FAMILY
HEALTH AND
EMERGENCY
GUIDE

FAMILY HEALTH AND EMERGENCY GUIDE

TIME LIFE BOOKS

LONDON

TIME®
LIFE
BOOKS

**PUBLISHED BY TIME-LIFE BOOKS,
LONDON 2000**

**ADAPTED FROM THE U.S. EDITION BY
ESSENTIAL BOOKS**

PROJECT EDITOR: EMMA DICKENS
TEXT EDITORS: ANNE CHARLISH, IAN PATEN

U.S. EDITORIAL STAFF

DIRECTOR OF EDITORIAL DEVELOPMENT: JENNIFER PEARCE
PROJECT EDITOR: ROBERT SOMERVILLE
SENIOR ART DIRECTOR: TINA TAYLOR
DEPUTY EDITORS: KRISTIN BAKER HANNEMAN,
TINA S. MCDOWELL
ADMINISTRATIVE EDITOR: JUDITH W. SHANKS
TEXT EDITORS: GLEN RUH, JIM WATSON
ASSOCIATE EDITORS/RESEARCH AND WRITING: NANCY
BLODGETT, KRISTIN DITTMAN, STEPHANIE SUM-
MERS HENKE, JENNIFER I. VERMILLION
TECHNICAL ART ASSISTANT: DANA R. MAGSUMBOLTT
PICTURE CREDITS: ALL ILLUSTRATIONS IN THIS BOOK WERE
CREATED BY TOTALLY INCORPORATED BY ROXANNA
DRAKE, CAROL HILLIARD, LESLIE LIEN, PETER
MALAMAS, TIPY TAYLOR, AND PATRICK WILSON

The textual and visual
decriptions of medical
conditions and treatment
options in this book should
be considered as a reference
source only; they are
not intended to be a
substitute for a healthcare
practitioner's diagnosis,
advice, and treatment.
Always consult your
doctor or a qualified
practitioner for proper
medical care.

Before using any drug or
natural medicine mentioned
in this book, be sure to
check with your healthcare
practitioner, and check
the product packaging or
other reliable source of
information for any
warnings or cautions. You
should keep in mind that
herbal remedies are not as
strictly regulated as drugs.

TABLE OF CONTENTS

INTRODUCTION

Whenever illnesses and emergencies strike, you're called upon to make critical medical decisions. You need to know the differences between situations that need immediate professional attention and those you can treat at home. You need to understand when a symptom is just an annoyance and when it may be an indication of something more serious.

In the context of the many treatment options available, these pages offer clear, concise information on the health problems you and your family are most likely to face. You'll be guided through the causes, symptoms, and methods of healing for each of the conditions. For any given ailment, conventional therapeutic approaches represent the best of modern medical science and mainstream medical practices. Alternative therapies also stand on extensive evidence of their benefits—even if those benefits sometimes defy scientific understanding.

In the end, the best choices will be those you make in conjunction with your healthcare practitioner. With this handy reference, you'll have the information you need to help make those decisions, and will be prepared to react quickly and effectively when you or someone you love is ill.

GUIDE TO COMPLEMENTARY THERAPIES

The world of medicine can seem overwhelmingly complex, with numerous fields of specialization divided between two broad sectors, generally called conventional and complementary. The distinction between the two approaches to medicine is best understood in terms of basic perceptions of health. Conventional medicine typically views health as an absence of disease. Among the key tools for healing are drugs, surgery, and radiation. Complementary medicine, by contrast, tends to view health as a balance of body systems—a principle called holism, meaning 'state of wholeness'. Any disharmony is thought to stress the body and perhaps lead to sickness. To fight disease, complementary medicine uses a wide range of therapies to bolster the body's own defences and restore balance. The following is an introduction to some of the most common complementary therapies.

ACUPRESSURE

This therapy involves pressing points on the body with fingers or hands to alter the internal flow of a supposed vital force or energy called chi (pronounced 'chee'), strengthening it, calming it, or removing a blockage of the flow. Acupressure is one of a number of treatment methods regularly used in traditional Chinese medicine, or TCM, a system of healthcare that originated in China thousands of years ago and is still widely practised in Asian countries today.

According to TCM, acupressure points are aligned along 14 bodily meridians, or pathways *(illustration, pages 138-139)*. Some well-controlled studies suggest that acupressure can be effective for a number of health problems, including nausea, pain, and stroke-related weakness. A single point may be pressed for relief from a particular symptom or condition; or to promote overall well-being of the body, a series of points can be worked on in a specific order. Acupressure may be practised at home.

The risks of acupressure are minimal, provided certain cautions are observed. During pregnancy, the points designated Spleen 6 and Large Intestine 4 should never be used; avoid the abdominal area entirely, if possible. Never apply pressure to open wounds, varicose veins, tumours, inflamed or infected skin, sites of recent surgery, or areas where a broken bone is suspected.

ACUPUNCTURE

Acupuncture, like acupressure, is based on the traditional Chinese theory of meridians—energy pathways that are believed to run through the body, carrying the vital force or energy called chi. In this therapy, the flow of chi is controlled by the insertion of hair-thin needles at specific points—the same meridian-aligned ones used in acupressure *(illustration, pages 8-9)*. Unlike acupressure, acupuncture must be performed by a trained practitioner.

In addition to (or sometimes instead of) inserting needles, acupuncturists may opt for a treatment called moxibustion. This consists of applying heat directly above acupuncture points by means of small bundles of smouldering herbs.

The ability of acupuncture to relieve pain in many patients is well documented, and the physical basis of the pain relief has been demonstrated through laboratory tests on animals; acupuncture releases endorphins and other forms of neurotransmitters that serve as the body's natural painkillers. Along with its pain-controlling benefits, acupuncture has been found effective in stroke rehabilitation and in providing relief from nausea.

AROMATHERAPY

In aromatherapy, the essential oils of plants are used to promote relaxation and help relieve the symptoms of certain ailments. Essential oils are concentrated fragrant extracts, cold-pressed or steam-distilled from blossoms, leaves, or roots. The oils are diluted with 'carrier' oils, such as almond or soy, and can be applied through massage, mixed with water and used as compresses on the skin, added to a bath, or diffused into the air and inhaled. Essential oils should never be ingested; one drop of oil can be equivalent to an ounce or more of a whole plant. Taken internally, the oils of some plants are toxic, and can even be fatal.

Aromatherapists believe that the properties of the oils have a soothing effect on the brain's limbic system, which is involved in memory, emotion, and hormone control. However, critics of aromatherapy suggest that the relaxation attributed to the oils may actually be due to their application by massage, hot baths, and other pleasant methods.

BODY WORK

Body work is an umbrella term for the many techniques that promote relaxation and treat ailments (especially those of the musculoskeletal system) through lessons in proper movement, postural re-education, exercise, massage, and other forms of bodily manipulation. Some types of body work—including massage, Chi Kung, reflexology, shiatsu, and t'ai chi—can be practised at home. Others may require the guidance of a trained professional. Forms of body work include the following:

◆ **The Alexander technique** focuses on correcting habitual posture and movement patterns that are believed to damage or impair the body's functioning.

◆ **Chi kung**, an ancient Chinese discipline, emphasizes breathing, meditation, and stationary and moving exercises to enhance the flow of energy or chi (sometimes also spelled 'qi') through the body.

◆ **The Feldenkrais method** is performed by a trained practitioner, during which verbally directed exercises, touch, and movement are used to teach new patterns in order to improve posture, movement, and breathing.

◆ **Massage** includes an assortment of manual therapies that manipulate the soft tissues of the body in order to reduce tension and stress, increase circulation, help to eliminate toxins, aid the healing of muscle and other soft-tissue injuries and control pain.

◆ **Reflexology** involves the manipulation of specific areas on the feet—and sometimes the hands—to bring the body into balance. According to reflexologists, distinct regions of the feet correspond to particular organs or body systems, and the stimulation of the appropriate region is intended to eliminate energy blockages thought to produce pain or disease. The arrangement of reflexology areas on the feet mirrors the organization of the body to the extent that organs on the right side of the body are represented on the right foot, and so with the left.

◆ **Rolfing** is based on the belief that proper alignment of the various parts of the body is necessary for physical and emotional health. The method uses deep massage and movement exercises to loosen or release adhesions in the fascia—the connective tissue covering muscles—in an effort to bring the body back into correct alignment.

◆ **Shiatsu**, a technique similar to acupressure, uses finger and thumb pressure on precise body points to encourage the proper flow of chi—or ki, as the Japanese call it—a vital force or energy believed to circulate through the body.

◆ **T'ai chi,** one style of qigong, is a martial art involving meditation and slow, flowing self-guided movements that follow set forms.

CHINESE HERBS

The use of herbs, along with acupuncture and acupressure, is a major part of the system of traditional Chinese medicine, or TCM. Doctors of TCM are usually titled 'licensed', or 'certified', acupuncturist, and they prescribe herbal combinations according to complex rules of diagnosis, which are intended to help the body correct imbalances of energies.

Chinese herbs can be prepared in numerous ways: steeped in hot water to make a tea or infusion; boiled to produce a stronger solution called a decoction; used to make powders, pills, or syrups that may all be taken internally; and fashioned into plasters or poultices that are applied to the skin. Treatments should be prescribed and monitored by a trained practitioner, because some Chinese herbs can be toxic in large doses. Some should be used with caution during pregnancy.

CHIROPRACTIC

Chiropractic is based on the idea that the human body has an innate self-healing ability. According to chiropractic theory, the nervous system plays a significant role in maintaining health. But problems in the joints are believed to interfere with proper functioning of the nervous system, and, as a result, the body's ability to maintain optimal health is diminished. Chiropractors seek to bring the body back into balance through manual manipulation of the spine and other joints and muscles, allowing the neuromusculoskeletal system to function smoothly.

Although chiropractic is categorized as complementary medicine, it has gained a degree of acceptance, in part because of a number of studies that have shown it to be effective in treating problems such as acute lower-back pain.

HERBAL THERAPIES

Herbal medicines are prepared from a variety of plant materials—leaves, stems, roots, bark, and so on. They usually contain many biologically active ingredients and are used primarily for treating mild or chronic ailments. Herbs can be prepared at home, using either fresh or dried ingredients. Herbal teas and infusions can be steeped to varying strengths. Roots, bark, or other plant parts can be boiled into strong solutions called decoctions. Honey or sugar can be added to infusions and decoctions to make syrups. Herbal remedies can also be purchased in the form of pills, capsules, or powders, or in more concentrated liquid forms called extracts and tinctures. They can be applied topically in creams or ointments, soaked into cloths and used as compresses, or applied directly to the skin as poultices.

Herbal remedies come in unpredictable strengths; the amount of the active ingredients varies greatly, depending on whether more than one species of the herb is used and how and when the herb is gathered and prepared. Because some herbs can be toxic or carcinogenic, all herbs should be used under the guidance of a herbalist or a healthcare practitioner familiar with herbal medicine.

HOMEOPATHY

Homeopathy is based on the idea that 'like cures like'; that is, substances that cause certain symptoms in a healthy person can also cure those same symptoms in someone who is sick.

The majority of homeopaths practise 'constitutional' homeopathy, based on the idea that each person's constitution—or mental, physical, and emotional makeup—may need to be treated along with any specific ailments. Classically, only one homeopathic medicine is used at a time. An extensive patient history is taken and the patient's physical and psychological symptoms are observed, then an initial prescription is made. If the medication does not have the desired effect or if the symptoms persist, a second analysis is done and a second prescription is given. This process continues until the correct medication for the underlying ailment is found. Constitutional treatment is generally used for chronic problems; acute, or short-term, ailments are usually treated with remedies specific to the illness.

Recently, over-the-counter combination homeopathic remedies have become available for a wide variety of ailments. These products contain several of the most common remedies for a particular problem and can be useful for self-treatment of minor conditions. For prolonged or serious illness, a professional homeopath can prescribe specific single remedies.

Homeopathic practitioners may have prior medical training, such as a degree in medicine, osteopathy, or naturopathic medicine.

MIND/BODY MEDICINE

This umbrella term covers activities and therapies that focus on the interrelationship of mind and body; the goal in all forms of mind/body medicine is to address particular disorders and promote overall health by combining both mental and physical approaches. Yoga, for example, involves both physical movement and a meditative state of mind, and may serve the dual purpose of improving a person's physical condition and combating emotional problems such as depression and anxiety. As noted below, the two-way connection between mind and body is exploited in many ways to influence the hormonal, nervous, and immune systems.

◆ **Biofeedback** uses computerized machines to measure and display body functions and states such as heart rate, skin temperature, muscle tension, and brain activity. By monitoring these functions through stages of rest and activity, patients are able to see how and why they change, and eventually can learn to control them.

◆ **Guided imagery** teaches patients to imagine scenarios that may help influence certain physiological conditions. A cancer patient, for example, may imagine a tumour dissolving under an attack by immune system 'bullets.'

◆ **Meditation** includes a number of different Asian and Western practices. All share the basic characteristics of sitting or resting quietly, often with the eyes closed, and performing mental exercises designed to relax the body and focus concentration.

◆ The **relaxation response** is a state of psychological and physiological rest characterized by lowered oxygen consumption and reduced heart rate. It can be induced by many different techniques, including **meditation, yoga, t'ai chi,** and **chi kung**. This deep relaxation can relieve stress.

◆ **Yoga** is a series of body positions and movements developed over thousands of years to calm the mind, relax the body, and ease the spirit. Meditation and breathing exercises lead into cycles of stretches and poses that may vary from session to session. Yoga can be learned and practised at home; however, modified movements may be required during pregnancy or if a person has a condition such as heart disease. A yoga specialist can recommend the appropriate adjustments.

NUTRITION AND DIET

Conventional and complementary practitioners alike acknowledge the importance of a healthy diet. Complementary practitioners, however, place more emphasis on dietary intervention in some conditions for which conventional medicine would resort first to drugs or even surgery.

Some diets, such as traditional Japanese and Mediterranean ones, contain small amounts of animal fat. Because they are low in saturated fats, these diets appear to protect against heart disease and some forms of cancer. Vegetarian diets have been shown to lower blood pressure and reduce the risk of cardiovascular disease and some cancers. Particular foods may be beneficial: garlic, for example, is said to reduce cholesterol levels and protect against some forms of cancer.

Vitamins and mineral supplements figure in the dietary recommendations of many therapies. Although some vitamins, such as A and D, are fat-soluble and can reach toxic levels in the body if not carefully monitored, others, such as vitamin C, are water-soluble and are not stored; any bodily excess is usually excreted. Generally, vitamins and minerals are recommended for daily use as a preventive measure.

OSTEOPATHY

Osteopathy focuses on correcting structural problems in the musculoskeletal system to improve overall bodily functioning. To restore structural balance and thus help a patient regain health, an osteopathic physician will combine manipulation of the joints, physical therapy, and instruction in proper posture. Because osteopathic care is holistic, or targeted at the whole body, the doctor also considers psychological factors, lifestyle, and diet in addressing an illness and maintaining health.■

EMERGENCIES/
FIRST AID ▶

What to Do in an Emergency

1 Telephone 999, or tell someone nearby to do so.

2 Check the victim's ABCs *(right)*.

3 Stop any severe bleeding *(page 14)*.

4 Prevent shock *(page 41)*.

5 Try to determine what happened. Look around the scene for any clues, such as an open container of a poisonous chemical.

The Recovery Position

Placing an unconscious victim who is breathing in the recovery position will keep the airway open. CAUTION: Do not place the victim in this position if you suspect a neck or back injury.

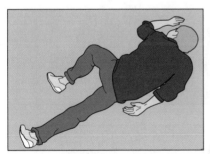

Support the victim's head and roll him onto his stomach. Bend the victim's arm and knee that are closest to you. Carefully tilt back the head so the airway remains open.

Checking the ABCs:
AIRWAY, BREATHING, CIRCULATION

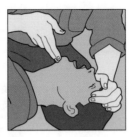

A

OPENING THE VICTIM'S AIRWAY. Gently tilt back the victim's head and lift the chin. CAUTION: If you suspect a head, neck, or back injury, just lift the chin.

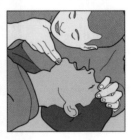

B

LOOKING, LISTENING, AND FEELING FOR BREATHING. Look for the victim's chest to rise. Put your ear to the victim's mouth, and listen and feel for exhaled air; chest movement alone might not mean breathing.

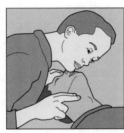

C

CHECKING FOR A PULSE. Gently press two fingers, not your thumb, in the depression on the side of the victim's neck, next to the Adam's apple, and feel for a pulse.

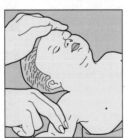

CHECKING FOR AN INFANT'S PULSE (UP TO 1 YEAR OLD). Gently press two fingers, not your thumb, on the inside of the infant's arm between the elbow and shoulder, and feel for a pulse. If you do not feel a pulse, listen for a heartbeat.

BLEEDING

IMPORTANT!

◆ If the bleeding is severe, telephone 999.

◆ For specific bleeding sites, see also Ear Emergencies *(page 24)*, Eye Emergencies *(page 28)*, or Nose Emergencies *(page 38)*.

CAUTION: If you suspect a head, neck, or back injury, see page 32.

1 **Lay the victim flat on his back.** Raise the victim's feet several centimetres. If possible, elevate the wound above heart level.

2 **Check the victim's ABCs** *(page 13)*. **If the victim is not breathing or does not have a pulse or heartbeat, begin CPR** *(pages 16-17)*.

3 **Remove any visible objects from the wound.** CAUTION: Do not remove any object or pull on any clothing that is stuck in the wound. Do not probe the wound or disturb it in any way.

4 **Apply direct pressure to the wound with a clean cloth or your hand.** If blood seeps through the cloth, do not remove it; put another cloth on top and keep pressing. You may need to apply firmer pressure if blood continues to seep through. For an embedded object, put pressure around the wound, not on the object.

5 **If the bleeding does not stop, apply pressure to an arterial pressure point.** Keep direct pressure on the wound as you press the arterial point. Do not apply pressure to arteries leading to the head or neck unless bright red blood is spurting from an injured neck artery.

6 **When the bleeding stops, apply a bandage.** Do not remove any cloths placed on the wound to help stop the bleeding; place a clean cloth over the wound. If there is an object embedded in the wound, bandage around it to support it.

7 **Keep the victim calm and still.**

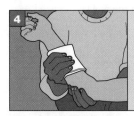

Applying direct pressure. Use a clean cloth, or your hand alone if necessary, to put pressure directly on the wound. Hold the edges of flesh together.

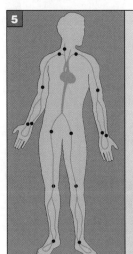
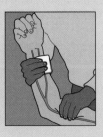

Applying pressure to an arterial pressure point. Apply pressure with your fingers held flat against the arterial pressure point that is closest to the wound, between it and the heart.

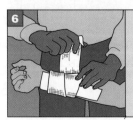

Bandaging a wound. Wrap a bandage or a clean cloth around the wound; tie it in place.

BURNS

◆ Telephone 999 if the burns involve more than one body part or the face, neck, hands, feet, or genitals, or if the victim has trouble breathing. Call if the victim is a child or is elderly.

◆ Telephone 999 if the burns are caused by chemicals. See the box below.

◆ If you suspect that the victim has been electrocuted, see Electric Shock (page 25).

◆ If the victim has a chemical burn in the eye, see Eye Emergencies (page 28).

◆ If the victim spilled a chemical that caused the skin to freeze, give first aid for chemical burns, then give first aid for frostbite (page 35).

◆ If the victim spilled a chemical that was absorbed through the skin without burning it, see Poisoning (page 39).

CAUTION: If you suspect a head, neck, or back injury, see page 32.

1 **Remove the victim from the cause of the burns.**

2 **Remove any clothing or jewellery from the burned area.** CAUTION: Do not remove any hot or smouldering clothing that is dry or is stuck to the burned skin. Do not breathe or cough on the burned skin.

3 **Cover small burns with wet cloths.** If the burned area is smaller than the size of the victim's chest, loosely cover it with a sheet or towel that has been soaked in cold water, or hold the burned skin under cold running water for 20 minutes. CAUTION: Do not place ice on the burned skin. Do not break any blisters. If the burned area is larger than the size of the victim's chest, do not apply water or cover the burn.

4 **Separate burned fingers or toes.** If fingers or toes have been burned, gently place dry cloth dressings between them. CAUTION: Do not use cotton or any adhesive bandages.

5 **Loosely cover the burned skin with a clean, dry cloth.** If fluid oozes through the cloth, place another cloth over it. CAUTION: Do not spread any ointments, lotions, butter, baking soda, or ice on the burn.

6 **Elevate a burned arm or leg above the level of the victim's heart.**

DEEP BURNS

For deep burns (indicated by charred or white skin), you should also check the victim's ABCs (page 13).

CLOTHING ON FIRE

1 **Lay the person on the ground so the burning clothing is on top.**
2 **Smother the flames with a blanket, coat, or any other cloth that is nearby and handy.** Direct the flames away from the person's face, or **tell the victim to roll over slowly.**

CHEMICAL BURNS

SYMPTOMS

◆ Burn marks	◆ Blisters
◆ Headache	◆ Dizziness
◆ Breathing problems	◆ Abdominal pain
◆ Seizures	◆ Unconsciousness

1 **Remove the victim from the chemical.**
2 **Flush the burn with water and remove contaminated clothing.** Place the burned area under running water for at least 15 minutes to dilute the chemical. As you flush the burn, remove any jewellery or clothing that may have come in contact with the chemical. CAUTION: For a dry chemical, such as lime, brush off any particles before flushing with water.
3 **Check the victim's ABCs** (page 13).
4 **If the victim is not breathing or does not have a pulse or heartbeat, begin CPR** (pages 16-17).
5 **Cover the burn with a clean, dry cloth.**

CARDIAC AND RESPIRATORY ARREST

CPR

Treatment for cardiac or respiratory arrest is called cardiopulmonary resuscitation (CPR). The goals of CPR are to open the airway, re-establish breathing, and re-establish circulation. It is best to give CPR only if you have been trained in the procedure.

CAUTION: If you suspect a head, neck, or back injury, see page 32.

1 Lay the victim flat on his back.

2 Sweep the victim's mouth. CAUTION: If you see an object lodged in the victim's throat, do not try to retrieve it, as this might force the object farther down the airway; give first aid for choking *(page 20)*.

3 Open the victim's airway. Gently tilt back the victim's head and lift the chin.

4 Look, listen, and feel for breathing. Be sure to put your ear to the victim's mouth; chest movement alone might not mean breathing.

5 If the victim is not breathing, give breaths. Watch for the chest to rise with each breath; let the chest fall before you give the second breath. If the victim's chest does not rise, gently tilt his head farther back and try again to give two slow breaths. If the chest still does not rise, give first aid for choking *(page 20)*. CAUTION: If the head is tilted too far or not far enough, you may not successfully open the airway.

6 Check for a pulse.

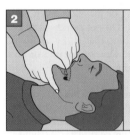

Finger sweep, adult. Hold the victim's tongue and lift the chin. Slide your index finger down the inside of the cheek and sweep out any loose objects.

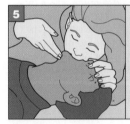

Giving breaths, adult. Pinch the nose shut and seal your lips tightly around the mouth. Give two slow breaths; remove your mouth between breaths.

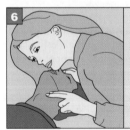

Checking the pulse, adult. Gently press two fingers, not your thumb, in the depression on the side of the victim's neck, next to the Adam's apple; feel for a pulse.

7 **If you feel no pulse, give chest compressions.** See the illustrations at right.

8 **Repeat steps 3, 4, and 5.** If the victim is an infant or a child younger than eight years old, give only one breath.

9 **Give chest compressions, breaths, and recheck for a pulse.** For an adult or child over eight years old, repeat a series of 15 chest compressions, followed by two breaths, 4 times; then recheck for a pulse. For an infant or a child younger than eight years old, repeat a series of 5 chest compressions, followed by one breath, 10 times; then recheck for a pulse. Repeat the series of chest compressions, breaths, and pulse checking until the victim has a pulse or begins to breathe on his own, or until medical help arrives.

10 **If the victim is not breathing but has a pulse, give breaths.** For an adult or child over eight years old, give 1 breath every five seconds. Check the pulse every 12 breaths. For a child between one and eight years old, give 1 breath every four seconds; check the pulse every 15 breaths. For an infant, give 1 breath every three seconds; check for a pulse or heartbeat every 20 breaths. Continue until help arrives.

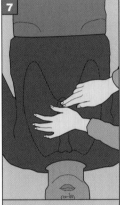

Placing your hands, adult. Place your middle finger in the notch where the ribs meet the bottom of the breastbone. Put your index finger next to and above your middle finger. Place the heel of your other hand next to and above your index finger. Remove your fingers and place that hand over your other hand; interlace your fingers and keep them up, off the chest.

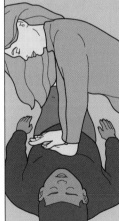

Giving chest compressions, adult. Position yourself so that your shoulders are directly over your hands; keep your arms straight. Press down forcefully to depress the victim's breastbone 4 to 5 centimetres. Release the pressure, but don't lift your hands off the chest. Give 15 chest compressions, at the count of 'one and two and three and....' CAUTION: Do not rock back and forth.

CONTINUED ▶

INFANT (UP TO 1 YEAR OLD)

SWEEP, BREATHS, PULSE

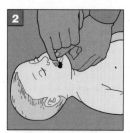

2

Finger sweep. Hold the tongue and lift the chin. Look in the mouth; if you can see an object and think you can easily remove it, slide your little finger down the inside of the cheek and sweep out the object.

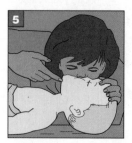

5

Giving breaths. Keep the chin lifted with one hand and seal your lips over the nose and mouth. First give two breaths, then one thereafter. Remove your mouth between breaths. Breathe forcefully but not so hard that air goes into the stomach.

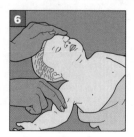

6

Checking the pulse. Gently press two fingers, not your thumb, on the inside of the infant's arm between the elbow and shoulder. If you do not feel a pulse, listen for a heartbeat.

CHEST COMPRESSIONS

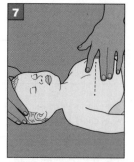

7

Placing your hands. Place your index finger just below an imaginary line between the nipples, in the center of the chest, on the breastbone. Place your two middle fingers next to and below your index finger, then lift your index finger. Use your free hand to help keep the infant's head tilted back.

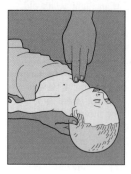

Giving chest compressions. Bend your elbow slightly and press straight down on your fingers, depressing the infant's breastbone 1¼ to 2½ centimetres. Release the pressure, but don't lift your fingers. Give five chest compressions, at the count of 'one two three....' CAUTION: Do not rock back and forth.

See pages 16-17 for complete instructions.

CHILD (BETWEEN 1 AND 8 YEARS OLD)

SWEEP, BREATHS, PULSE

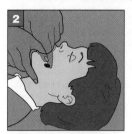

Finger sweep. Hold the victim's tongue and lift the chin. Slide your index finger down the inside of the cheek and sweep out any loose objects.

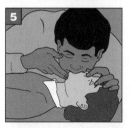

Giving breaths. Pinch the nose shut and seal your lips tightly around the mouth. Give two slow breaths initially; give one breath thereafter. Remove your mouth between breaths.

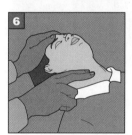

Checking the pulse. Gently press two fingers, not your thumb, in the depression on the side of the victim's neck, next to the Adam's apple, and feel for a pulse.

CHEST COMPRESSIONS

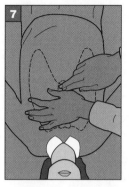

Placing your hands. Place two fingers of your right hand in the notch where the ribs meet the bottom of the breastbone. Place the heel of your left hand next to your right index finger, keeping your fingers off the child's chest. Now remove your left hand and put the heel of your right hand where the left hand was. Use your left hand to keep the child's head tilted back *(below)*.

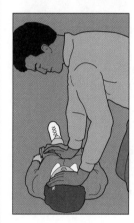

Giving chest compressions. Position yourself so that your shoulders are directly over the child's chest; keep your arm straight. Press down forcefully on your hand to depress the child's breastbone 2½ to 4 centimetres. Release the pressure, but don't lift your hand. Give five chest compressions, at the count of 'one and two and three and....' CAUTION: Do not rock back and forth.

See pages 16-17 for complete instructions.

CHOKING

IMPORTANT!

◆ If you suspect that an object is caught in a victim's throat and he cannot cough, breathe, speak, or cry, call 999 or tell someone nearby to do so. Begin first-aid treatment for choking *(below)*. If you are the victim, see the box below, right. If the victim is an infant (up to one year old), see the box on page 22.

◆ If you suspect that an object is caught in a victim's throat but he is able to cough, breathe, talk, or cry, do not intervene. But be prepared to act if the situation worsens.

CAUTION: If you suspect a head, neck, or back injury, see page 32.

1 **Do not try to retrieve an object lodged in the victim's throat.** This might force the object farther down the airway.

2 **Give abdominal thrusts (the Heimlich manoeuvre).** Continue giving abdominal thrusts until the object is dislodged or until the victim loses consciousness. CAUTION: If the victim is pregnant or obese, place your fist on the middle of the victim's breastbone; do not place your hands on the ribs or on the lower edge of the breastbone.

3 **If the victim loses consciousness, lay him flat on his back.**

4 **Sweep the victim's mouth.** CAUTION: Remember, do not try to retrieve an object lodged in the victim's throat.

5 **Open the victim's airway.** Gently tilt back the victim's head and lift the chin.

6 **Look, listen, and feel for breathing.** Be sure to put your ear to the victim's mouth; chest movement alone might not mean breathing. If the victim is breathing, give first aid for unconsciousness *(page 37)*.

7 **Breathe twice into the victim's mouth.** Watch for the victim's chest to rise with each breath; let the chest fall before you give the next breath. If the victim's chest does not rise with each breath, gently tilt the head farther back and try again to give two slow breaths.

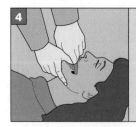

Abdominal thrust. Place your arms around the victim's waist. Make a fist with one hand and place it in the middle of the victim's abdomen, just above the navel and below the ribs. Hold your fist with your other hand. Give quick, repeated thrusts, pushing inward and upward.

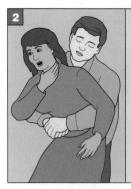

Finger sweep. Hold the victim's tongue and lift the chin. Slide your index finger down the inside of the cheek and sweep out any loose objects.

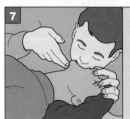

Breathe into the victim's mouth. Pinch the victim's nose shut and seal your lips tightly around the mouth. Give two slow breaths; remove your mouth between breaths.

8 If the victim's chest still does not rise, give five abdominal thrusts. CAUTION: Do not press to either side as you thrust.

9 Sweep the victim's mouth, make sure the airway is open, and breathe twice again into the victim's mouth.

10 If the victim's chest still does not rise, give abdominal thrusts, sweep the mouth, and give breaths. Give five abdominal thrusts. Sweep the victim's mouth, and give two slow breaths. Repeat this sequence of abdominal thrusts, sweeps of the mouth, and slow breaths until the object is dislodged or until medical help arrives.

11 If the object is dislodged but the victim is not breathing, begin CPR *(pages 16-17)*.

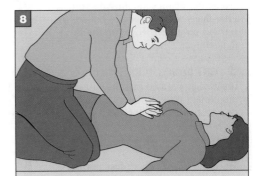

Abdominal thrust. Position the heel of one of your hands against the middle of the victim's abdomen, just above the navel and below the ribs. Place your other hand on top of the first. Give quick thrusts, pressing your hands inward and upward.

SELF

Give yourself abdominal thrusts until the object is dislodged. Get medical help to check for complications arising from either the choking episode or the first aid. CAUTION: If you feel or see an object lodged in your throat, do not try to retrieve it, as this might force the object farther down your airway.

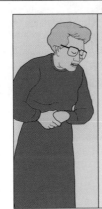

Abdominal thrust. Make a fist with one hand and place it in the middle of your abdomen, just above the navel and below the ribs. Hold your fist with your other hand. Keeping your elbows out, press your fist with a quick, upward thrust into your abdomen.

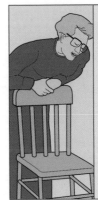

Abdominal thrust with the help of an object. Make a fist with one hand and place it in the middle of your abdomen, just above the navel and below the ribs. Bend over the back of a chair, a countertop, or some other firm, hard object and forcefully press it against your fist.

CONTINUED ▶

INFANT (UP TO 1 YEAR OLD)

1 **Give back blows and chest thrusts.** Give four back blows. If the object is not dislodged, give four chest thrusts. Repeat sets of four back blows and four chest thrusts until the object is dislodged or the infant loses consciousness.

2 **If the infant loses consciousness, sweep the infant's mouth with your little finger.** CAUTION: Do not try to retrieve an object lodged in the infant's throat.

3 **Give breaths.** If the infant isn't breathing, give two breaths into the mouth and nose. If the infant's chest does not rise with each breath, gently tilt the head farther back and try again to give two breaths.

4 **If the infant's chest does not rise with breaths, continue giving breaths, back blows, and chest thrusts and sweeps of the mouth.** Repeat a sequence of two breaths, four back blows, four chest thrusts, and a sweep of the mouth until the object is dislodged or until medical help arrives.

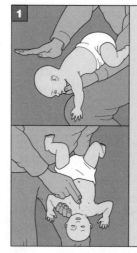

Back blow. Lay the infant facedown on your lower arm, supporting the head with your hand. Hold the chin between your index finger and thumb. Strike the back between the shoulder blades with the heel of your other hand.

Chest thrust. Turn the infant onto his back, with his head lower than the rest of his body. Place your index and middle fingers on the breastbone just below the nipples. Give quick thrusts.

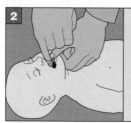

Finger sweep. Hold the infant's tongue and lift the chin. If you see an object and believe that you can easily remove it, slide your little finger down the inside of the cheek and sweep the object out.

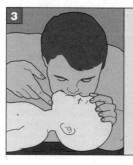

Breathe into the infant's mouth. Keep the head tilted with one hand and the chin lifted with your other. Tightly seal your lips around the mouth and nose. Give two breaths; remove your mouth between breaths. Breathe forcefully but not so hard that air goes into the infant's stomach.

DROWNING OR NEAR-DROWNING

CAUTION: If you suspect a head, neck, or back injury, see page 32.

1 **Pull the victim to safety.** CAUTION: Be careful if you stretch out your arm or leg to the victim; the victim may inadvertently pull you into the water. Try to keep the victim's head, neck, and back aligned as you pull him to shore; if possible, slip a board under his back to tow him or to carry him out of the water.

2 **Check the victim's ABCs** *(page 13)*. **If the victim is not breathing or does not have a pulse or heartbeat, begin CPR** *(pages 16-17)*.

3 **Place the victim in the recovery position** *(page 13)*. CAUTION: Do not place the victim in the recovery position if you suspect a neck or back injury, perhaps caused by a diving accident.

4 **Remove any wet clothing and cover the victim with a coat, blanket, or dry clothing.**

5 **Keep the victim still and quiet while you wait for medical help to arrive.**

WATER RESCUE

Unconscious victim. If possible, wade out and tow the victim face uppermost to shore; be careful of strong currents. If the water is too deep for wading, look for a boat to use to get to the victim. If there is no boat nearby and you are a strong swimmer, swim out to the victim and tow him face up to shore. Otherwise, get help.

Conscious victim. Pull the drowning victim to safety with the help of a stick, oar, rope and life ring, towel, or nearby boat. If necessary, wade toward the victim, but be careful of strong currents. CAUTION: Do not swim out to the victim, unless you have been trained in water rescues.

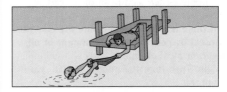

ICE RESCUE

Unconscious victim. If you can't reach the victim, tie a rope to a tree and then around your waist; slide on your belly to the victim. Otherwise, form a human chain with rescuers lying flat on the ice, and pull the victim to shore. CAUTION: Stay as far away as possible from the break in the ice.

Conscious victim. Tell the victim not to climb out but to hang on to the edge of the ice. Pull the victim out with the help of a big stick, rope, or ladder. Or form a human chain with rescuers lying flat on the ice.

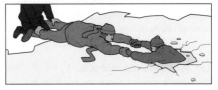

EAR EMERGENCIES

Foreign Objects

1 **Shake the object out.** Tilt the victim's head so that the affected ear is near the ground. Ask the victim to shake his head, or shake it for him. CAUTION: Do not hit the victim's head to try to free the object.

2 **Pick the object out.** If the object does not fall out, look into the ear. If you can see the object and it is pliable but is not a live insect, try to remove it with tweezers. CAUTION: Never poke at an object. Do not try to pick out a hard object such as a bean or a bead.

3 **If there is a live insect inside the ear, kill the insect by pouring a small amount of oil, vinegar, or alcohol onto it.** This will help alleviate pain. Then float the insect out with warm, not hot, oil.

4 **If the object is securely lodged in the ear,** take the victim to the nearest hospital.

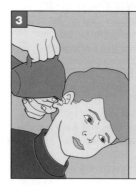

Floating an insect out of the ear. Tilt the victim's head so that the affected ear is toward the sky. Gently pull the victim's earlobe backward and upward, and pour a little warm mineral, olive, or baby oil into the ear. This should float the insect out of the ear.

Blood or Other Fluids from inside the Ear

1 **Loosely cover the ear with a clean cloth and tape the cloth in place.** CAUTION: Do not try to stop the drainage. Do not try to clean the ear.

2 **Lay the victim flat on his back.** CAUTION: If you suspect a head, neck, or back injury, see page 32.

ELECTRIC SHOCK

CAUTION: If you suspect a head, neck, or back injury, see page 32.

1 **Stop the flow of electricity.** Switch off supply at plug switch. Unplug the electrical appliance or turn off the house's main power switch. If you are not able to do this, separate the victim from the live current, using a broom with a wooden handle, or a wooden chair, for example. CAUTION: Do not touch the victim's skin while he is still touching the live current. Do not touch the electrical wire.

2 **Check the victim's ABCs** *(page 13).* **If the victim is not breathing or does not have a pulse or heartbeat, begin CPR** *(pages 16-17).*

3 **Check for and treat any other serious injury.** Treat any entry and exit burns *(page 15).*

4 **Make the victim comfortable.** Cover the victim with a coat or blanket. Do not place a pillow under the head; this might cause the airway to become blocked.

SYMPTOMS

◆ Burn marks on mouth or skin
◆ Tingling sensation
◆ Dizziness
◆ Feeling a severe jolt
◆ Muscle pains
◆ Bleeding
◆ Headache
◆ Unconsciousness

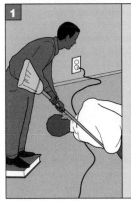

Separating the victim from the current. Stand on a pile of clothes, a book, or a piece of wood; make sure you are not standing in a pool of water. Use a dry, nonconductive material such as a wooden broom handle or a wood chair to separate the victim from the live current.

EMERGENCY CHILDBIRTH

Preparing the Mother

1 **Make the mother comfortable.** Place her on a large, flat area with pillows or other comfortable, supportive materials. Put a clean sheet or newspapers under her. Make sure she is warm. Help her remove any clothing below her belly.

2 **Keep the mother calm.** The mother may be in great pain; tell her to take deep, slow breaths.

3 **Wash your hands with soap and water.** Scrub under your fingernails with soap and water, and remove all of your jewellery.

The Delivery

1 **Bloodstained fluid will appear.** It is normal for there to be some bloodstained fluid; do not be alarmed. CAUTION: Get immediate medical help if the mother bleeds more than 1 to 2 cups of blood before, during, or after delivery.

2 **Support the baby as he emerges.** The baby will be slippery; you may want to use a clean, dry towel to hold him. CAUTION: Do not pull on the baby.

3 **Make sure the umbilical cord is not around the baby's neck.** If the umbilical cord is wrapped around the baby's neck, tell the mother not to push for a moment or two while you hook your finger underneath the cord and gently slip it over the baby's head.

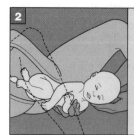

Support the baby. Most babies emerge headfirst. Support his head, and the rest of his body, as he emerges. He will naturally turn to one side and the rest of his body will follow.

4 **The baby's shoulder may get stuck.** If a shoulder seems stuck, gently press just above the mother's pubic hair or raise her legs up; tell her to push hard.

5 **The baby may still be in the amniotic sac.** If this is the case, tear the sac open.

6 **The baby's head may not emerge first.** If this happens, gently press just above the mother's pubic hair. Note the time. Support the baby's body as he emerges. If the head is not delivered within three minutes, lift the baby's body to expose his face so he can breathe. Tell the mother to keep pushing. CAUTION: Do not pull the baby out of the vagina.

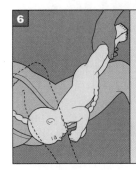

Let a breech baby breathe. Lift the baby's body upward until you can see his face. Clean the baby's mouth and nose with a clean, dry towel.

After the Birth

1 **Help the baby begin to breathe.** Hold the baby so fluids drain from his mouth and nose. Clean his mouth and nose with a clean, dry towel. If he is not breathing, hold him so his head is lower than his feet and tap his soles. Immediately rub his back. If this doesn't work, begin CPR *(pages 16-17).*

2 **Dry and wrap the baby.** Use a clean, dry towel; do not wash off any white, waxy material on his body. Wrap him in a clean, dry towel.

3 **Tie a string around the umbilical cord.**

4 **Save the placenta.** The mother will usually expel the placenta within 30 minutes. Place it in a container to give to medical personnel. If it is not entirely expelled within 30 minutes, get immediate medical help. Do not pull on the umbilical cord or try to get the placenta out.

5 **Massage the mother's lower abdomen.** After the placenta is expelled, rub the mother's lower abdomen to help control any bleeding.

6 **Keep the mother and baby warm until medical help arrives.**

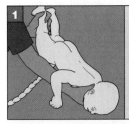

Drain the baby's fluids. Hold the baby so his head is lower than his feet and turn his head sideways.

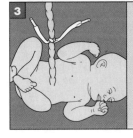

Tie off the umbilical cord. Use a string or shoelace and tie it tightly around the umbilical cord at least 10 centimetres away from the baby's navel. CAUTION: Do not use thread to tie the umbilical cord.

EYE EMERGENCIES

Foreign Objects

CAUTION: Do not touch or attempt to remove anything embedded in the eye. If the object is large, such as a pen, place a paper cup over the eye so that it supports the object; you may need to punch a hole in the cup. Tape the cup in place. Cover the victim's other eye with a clean cloth to help keep the injured eye from moving. If the object is small, cover both eyes with a clean cloth and loosely tie it in place.

1 Wash your hands with soap and water.

2 **Look for the object.** Ask the victim to slowly roll his eyes as you look for the object. CAUTION: Do not let the victim rub his eye.

3 **Cause tears to form in the eye.** If you see the object, gently pull the upper eyelid down over the lower eyelid. This will cause tears, which may wash the object out.

4 **Remove a visible object.** If the object does not wash out with tears, flush it out with running water or lift it off with a clean, damp cloth. Alternatively, the victim can open his eyes underwater in a bowl of fresh tap water. Once the object is out, the victim should take out any contact lenses. CAUTION: Do not use tissue or cotton to lift off the object. Do not attempt to lift off an object that is on the victim's iris or pupil.

5 **Remove an object from the lower eyelid.** If you see the object on the lower eyelid, flush it out with water or lift it off with a clean, damp cloth. Once the object is out, the victim should take out any contact lenses.

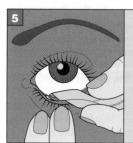

Lifting an object off the lower eyelid. Tell the victim to look up, and gently pull down the lower eyelid. Lift the object off the eye with a clean, damp cloth. CAUTION: Do not use tissue or cotton to lift off the object.

6 **Remove an object off the upper eyelid.** If you do not see the object on the eye or inside the lower eyelid, lift the victim's upper eyelid. If you see the object on the upper eyelid, flush it out with water or lift it off with a clean, damp cloth. Once the object is out of the eye, flip the upper eyelid back into place. The victim should now take out any contact lenses. CAUTION: Do not use tissue or cotton to lift off the object.

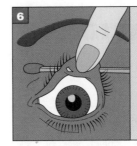

Raising the upper eyelid. Tell the victim to look down. Place a cotton wool bud, matchstick, or coffee stirrer across the upper eyelid. Hold the victim's upper eyelashes and eyelid, and fold the upper eyelid over the matchstick.

7 **If necessary, cover both eyes and get medical help.** If you cannot find or remove the object, or if the victim is in pain or has difficulty seeing after you've removed the object, cover both eyes with a clean cloth and tie it in place. Take the victim to the nearest hospital.

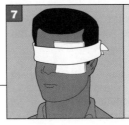

Covering both eyes. Place a clean cloth over the injured eye. Wrap another clean cloth around the victim's head so that it covers both eyes; tie it in place.

Chemical in the Eye

CAUTION: Immediately start flushing the eye with water, and make sure that the water is getting underneath both eyelids. Do not put anything other than water in the eye. Do not let the victim rub his eye.

1 **Flush the eye with water.** See the illustration at right. If you cannot get the victim to a tap, keep flushing the eye with glasses of water for 15 minutes, making sure that the water flows across the eye away from the inner corner.

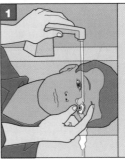

Flushing the eye. Hold the person's open eye under running water from a tap for at least 15 minutes. The water should run from the inside of the eye to the outside. If both eyes are affected, let the water run over both eyes.

2 **Ask the victim to remove his contact lenses, if he is wearing any.**

3 **Cover the eye.** After flushing the eye, cover it with a clean cotton cloth. Then tie a bandage over both eyes; this will help inhibit movement of the affected eye.

4 **Identify, if you can, the chemical that caused the burn.** At least be prepared to tell emergency medical personnel whether the chemical was wet or dry.

FRACTURES AND DISLOCATIONS

◆ Telephone 999.

◆ If you suspect that the victim has broken his neck or back, see Head, Neck, and Back Injuries *(page 32)*.

◆ If you suspect that the victim has broken his nose, see Nose Emergencies *(page 38)*.

SYMPTOMS

◆ Pain
◆ Misshapen body part
◆ Bruising
◆ Discoloration of skin
◆ Swelling
◆ Visible bone
◆ Numbness in limb
◆ Loss of function of joint, limb, or digit

CAUTION: If you suspect a head, neck, or back injury, see page 32.

1 **Check the victim's ABCs** *(page 13).* **If the victim is not breathing or does not have a pulse or heartbeat, begin CPR** *(pages 16-17).*

2 **Do not move the victim.** CAUTION: Do not move someone with an injured hip, pelvis, or upper leg unless it is absolutely necessary. If you must move him to safety, immobilize the victim's head between your arms, grab his clothes at his shoulders, and drag him.

3 **Check for and treat any other serious injuries.** CAUTION: If the victim is bleeding around or near a broken bone, do not wash or probe the wound. Place a clean cloth over the wound and tie a bandage over it.

4 **Immobilize the injured bone or joint.** If a finger or toe is broken, apply a cold compress to it and elevate it above the level of the victim's heart. Place a small cloth or piece of cotton between the injured digit and an uninjured one, and then tape them together. See the illustrations opposite for instructions on how to immobilize an injured leg or arm. CAUTION: Do not attempt to straighten or change the position of any misshapen bone or joint. When applying a sling or splint, do not cut off blood circulation to the injured limb. Do not tie the splint in place over the break.

IMMOBILIZING AN INJURED ARM

LOWER ARM, WRIST, OR HAND

STABILIZE THE INJURED ARM

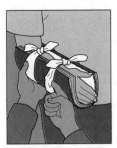

Stabilizing the arm. Support the injured bone or wrist with your hands, and place the lower arm at a right angle over the victim's chest. The victim's thumb should be pointing upward. Place the arm and wrist on a magazine or newspaper padded with a towel or pillow, and tie the magazine in place.

PLACE THE ARM IN A SLING

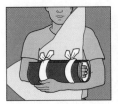

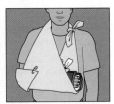

1 Position a cloth to be used as a sling. Locate a large piece of cloth or a long-sleeved shirt or sweater; fold the cloth in half, so it forms a triangle. Slide the cloth or shirt between the victim's arm and body, so the long side of the cloth or the shirt's top is closest to the uninjured arm.

2 Tie the cloth in place. Pull one end of the cloth behind the victim's neck; place the other half over the injured arm. Tie the sling over the shoulder of the uninjured side; fold over any extra material that is behind the elbow and pin it in place. Make sure the sling is snug but not tight.

UPPER ARM, SHOULDER, OR COLLARBONE

STABILIZE THE INJURED SHOULDER OR COLLARBONE

1 Support the injured bone or joint with your hands. Position the injured arm across the chest, thumb pointing up, and place it in a sling *(above)*.

2 Secure the sling in place. Tie a piece of cloth around the sling and the victim's chest and arm.

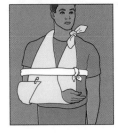

IMMOBILIZING AN INJURED LEG

LOWER LEG

SPLINT THE LOWER LEG

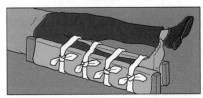

Using boards as a splint. Locate two long boards; one should extend from the victim's hip to the heel, and the second should stretch from the groin to the heel. Pad the boards with blankets or pillows, then place the boards so the padded side touches the injured leg. Tie the boards in place at the groin, thigh, knee, and ankle.

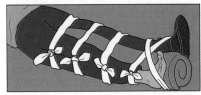

Using a blanket as a splint. If boards are unavailable, roll up a blanket, place it between the victim's legs, and tie the victim's legs together at the groin, thighs, knees, and ankles.

UPPER LEG OR HIP

SPLINT THE UPPER LEG OR HIP

CAUTION: Do not splint an injured upper leg or hip unless you have to move the victim. Do not tie the splint in place over the break.

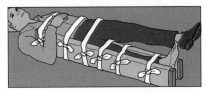

Using boards as a splint. Locate two long boards: one to extend from the victim's armpit to the heel, and the other from the groin to the heel. Pad the boards with blankets or pillows, then place the boards padded side in. Tie the boards in place at the chest, waist, groin, thigh, knee, and ankle.

31

HEAD, NECK, AND BACK INJURIES

CAUTION: Do not move the injured person unless it is absolutely necessary.

1 **Keep the victim calm and completely still.**

2 **Check the victim's ABCs** *(page 13)*. **If the victim is not breathing or does not have a pulse or heartbeat, begin CPR** *(pages 16-17)*. CAUTION: When opening the victim's airway, just lift the chin. If you need to place the victim on his back, support his head, neck, and back together and carefully roll him on to his back; make sure you keep the head, neck, and back aligned as you roll him. It is best to have at least one other person help you do this.

3 **Treat obvious injuries.**

4 **Make the victim comfortable.** Keep the victim warm, with a blanket or coat, until medical help arrives. CAUTION: Do not put a pillow under the head, as this might cause the airway to become blocked. Do not give him anything to eat or drink.

5 **Keep the airway open.** If the victim begins to choke or vomit or becomes unconscious, support his head, neck, and back together and carefully roll him on to his side. It is best to have someone else help you do this. CAUTION: Make sure that the victim's head and neck move with his body.

SYMPTOMS

Head Injuries

- Head wound
- Bruise or lump on scalp
- Bleeding from ear, nose, or mouth that is not due to injury to those areas
- Fluid draining from ear or nose
- Black eyes
- Bruise behind ear
- Headache, nausea, or vomiting
- Altered mental state
- Vision changes
- Slurred speech
- Drowsiness
- Irregular pulse
- Unconsciousness

Neck or Back Injuries

- Pain in back or neck
- Tingling sensation in arms or legs
- Loss of movement in arms or legs
- Loss of bladder or bowel control
- Odd position of head, neck, or back
- Unconsciousness

HEART ATTACK

SYMPTOMS

- Crushing or spreading chest pain that may radiate to one or both arms or to the neck or jaw
- Irregular heartbeat
- Difficulty in breathing
- Fear or anxiety
- Complaining of indigestion
- Dizziness
- Heavy sweating
- Nausea or vomiting
- Pale or bluish lips or fingernails
- Pale, bluish, or clammy skin
- Unconsciousness

CAUTION: If you suspect a head, neck, or back injury, see page 32.

1 Check the victim's ABCs *(page 13)*. If the victim is not breathing or does not have a pulse or heartbeat, begin CPR *(pages 16-17)*.

2 Make the victim comfortable and keep him calm. Loosen any tight clothing, especially around the victim's neck, chest, and waist. If the victim is unconscious, place him in the recovery position *(page 13)*. Keep the victim warm; if necessary, cover him with a blanket or additional clothing. Stroke the victim's forehead with a cool, wet cloth. CAUTION: Do not try to revive an unconscious victim by slapping or shaking him or throwing cold water on him. Do not give the victim anything to eat or drink.

3 Continue to monitor the victim's breathing and pulse, and if necessary, begin CPR.

HEATSTROKE AND HEAT EXHAUSTION

Heatstroke

Cool the victim. Quickly move the victim to a cooler site. Place cool, wet cloths on the forehead and torso, or wrap the victim in wet towels or sheets. Fan him with an electric fan, a hair dryer set on cold, or your hand. CAUTION: Do not use an alcohol rub to cool the victim; do not give him anything to eat or drink.

Heat Exhaustion

1 Move the victim to a cooler site.

2 Have the victim lie or sit down, and elevate his feet.

3 Cool the victim. Place cool, wet cloths on the forehead and torso, or wrap the victim in wet towels or sheets. Fan the victim with an electric fan, a hair dryer set on cold, or your hand. CAUTION: Do not use an alcohol rub to cool the victim.

4 Give the conscious victim a cool drink. If the victim is conscious and is able to swallow and breathe without difficulty, give him salt water (1 tsp salt mixed with just over 1 litre water) to sip. CAUTION: Do not force the victim to drink; do not give him anything that is alcoholic or caffeinated.

5 If the victim's condition does not improve, telephone 999.

IMPORTANT!

◆ If you suspect that the victim is suffering from heatstroke, telephone 999.

SYMPTOMS

Heatstroke

◆ Body temperature above 39°C (over 101°F)
◆ Flushed, dry, hot skin
◆ Constricted pupils
◆ Confusion
◆ Rapid pulse
◆ Seizures
◆ Unconsciousness

Heat Exhaustion

◆ Cool, clammy skin
◆ Excessive perspiration
◆ Dilated pupils
◆ Rapid pulse
◆ Headache
◆ Nausea or vomiting
◆ Abdominal or limb cramps
◆ Dizziness
◆ Sense of room rotating
◆ Unconsciousness

HYPOTHERMIA AND FROSTBITE

SYMPTOMS

Hypothermia

◆ Shivering
◆ Uncoordinated movements
◆ Drowsiness, weakness
◆ Unconsciousness
◆ Cardiac arrest

Frostbite

◆ Numb, cold skin
◆ Pink skin that becomes pale, and then later becomes blackened or hard and frozen
◆ Blisters

Hypothermia

CAUTION: If you suspect a head, neck, or back injury, see page 32.

1 Check the victim's ABCs *(page 13).* **If the victim is not breathing or does not have a pulse or heartbeat, begin CPR** *(pages 16-17).* CAUTION: Hypothermic victims often have very slow and weak pulses; therefore, take a little extra time and care to check for the pulse.

2 Gently take or lead the victim to shelter. Change the victim into dry clothing.

3 If medical help is unavailable, slowly rewarm the victim. Cover the head and neck. Use your own body heat, blankets, or aluminum foil to slowly warm the victim. Place warm compresses to the neck, chest, and groin. If the victim is conscious and can swallow, give warm, sweetened, nonalcoholic beverages to sip. CAUTION: Do not use any form of direct heat, such as an electric blanket, to warm the victim.

Frostbite

CAUTION: If there is any chance of the skin refreezing, do not thaw it. Move the victim out of the cold and wait for emergency help.

1 Move the victim to a nearby shelter. Remove any tight clothing or jewellery.

2 If you can keep the frostbitten skin warm and help will not arrive soon, slowly thaw the skin. Place frostbitten hands or feet in a bowl of warm, not hot, water for at least 30 minutes. Gently stir the water, and add warm water as it cools. Or soak a cotton cloth in warm water; resoak the cloth to keep it warm. If water is not available, use your own skin, blankets, or newspaper to warm the skin. CAUTION: Frostbitten skin may be permanently damaged if warmed too quickly; do not use direct heat, such as an electric blanket. Do not massage the skin.

3 Dry the thawed skin and keep it warm. Once the damaged skin is soft and sensation returns, place a clean, dry cloth over the skin; place clean, dry cloths between frostbitten toes and fingers. Wrap the skin with dry cloths in order to keep it warm.

4 Do not let the victim smoke or drink alcohol while you wait for medical help.

INTERNAL BLEEDING

SYMPTOMS

◆ Bruises
◆ Coughing or vomiting blood
◆ Rectal bleeding
◆ Vaginal (but not menstrual) bleeding
◆ Blood in urine
◆ Bleeding from the nose or ear
◆ Skull, chest, or abdominal wounds
◆ Dizziness
◆ Fainting
◆ Weak pulse
◆ Shortness of breath
◆ Shallow breathing
◆ Dilated pupils
◆ Pale, clammy skin
◆ Fits/convulsions

CAUTION: If you suspect a head, neck, or back injury, see page 32.

1 Check the victim's ABCs *(page 13)*. **If the victim is not breathing or does not have a pulse or heartbeat, begin CPR** *(pages 16-17)*. While you wait for medical help, periodically recheck the victim's ABCs.

2 **Keep the victim calm and still. Do not give him anything to eat or drink.**

3 **If the victim's arm or leg is swollen or mis-shapen, immobilize it** *(page 31)*.

4 **Begin treatment for shock** *(page 41)* **while you wait for medical help.**

LOSS OF CONSCIOUSNESS

CAUTION: If you suspect a head, neck, or back injury, see page 32.

1 **Check the victim's ABCs** *(page 13)*. **If the victim is not breathing or does not have a pulse or heartbeat, begin CPR** *(pages 16-17)*.

2 **Remove the victim from an injurious site.**

3 **Loosen any tight clothing, especially around the victim's neck.**

4 **Place the victim in the recovery position** *(page 13).*

5 **Keep the victim warm, with a blanket or coat, until medical help arrives.** Stroke the victim's forehead with a cool, wet cloth. CAUTION: Do not try to revive the victim by slapping or shaking him or throwing cold water on him. Do not place a pillow under the head, as this might cause the airway to become blocked.

NOSE EMERGENCIES

SYMPTOMS

Foreign Objects

♦ Irritation
♦ Difficulty breathing through nostril
♦ Foul odour from nose
♦ Foul-smelling discharge from nostril
♦ Bleeding from nostril

Nosebleed

♦ Bleeding from nostril
♦ Bleeding in the back of the throat
♦ Gagging
♦ Choking

Foreign Objects

CAUTION: Do not use tweezers or other tools to try to remove the object. Do not ask the victim to inhale sharply.

1 Ask the victim to try to blow out the object. Press the unaffected nostril with one finger; ask the victim to blow his nose. If the object is not dislodged, ask the victim to sniff some pepper to help him sneeze and blow the object out.

2 If the object is still not dislodged, take the victim to the nearest hospital.

Nosebleed

CAUTION: If your nose is misshapen or misaligned, or you have swelling, pain, or bruises around your eyes, your nose may be broken. Sit down and press a cold cloth against your nose. Ask someone to take you to the nearest hospital.

1 Sit down.

2 If there are clots of blood in your nose, try to blow them out, once.

3 Pinch your nose shut. Hold both nostrils, below the bridge, between your thumb and index finger for 10 minutes. Breathe through your mouth.

4 If the bleeding does not stop, place a cloth packing in the bleeding nostril. Roll a small, clean cloth and place it in the bleeding nostril; hold both nostrils between your thumb and index finger. CAUTION: Do not push the cloth too far into the nose; make sure that you will be able to pull it out.

5 Once the bleeding stops, place a cold cloth over your nose and face.

6 Remove the cloth packing in your nostril after 30 to 60 minutes. It is best to dampen the cloth before removing it. Do not blow or pick your nose, strain yourself, or bend over for 24 hours. Rub petroleum jelly inside the nostril to help prevent further bleeding or drying.

POISONING

CAUTION: If you suspect a head, neck, or back injury, see page 32.

1 **Check the victim's ABCs** *(page 13)*. **If the victim is not breathing or does not have a pulse or heartbeat, begin CPR** *(pages 16-17)*.

2 **Try to identify the poison.** If possible, ask the victim what he swallowed or inhaled. Otherwise, look around for any open or nearby containers of chemicals or for any plants or household items that the victim may have swallowed; sniff the air for unusual odours.

3 **Telephone 999, or National Poisons Information Service on 0870 600 6266, or NHS Direct 0845 4647.** Tell emergency personnel what chemical, plant, or household item the victim swallowed. Wait for instructions as to how to proceed.

4 **Follow the instructions given by the Poisons Information Service or by 999 personnel.** Depending on the poison, you may be instructed to induce vomiting, to give milk or water to drink, or to give activated charcoal. CAUTION: Do not try to induce vomiting unless told to do so; do not induce vomiting if it has been more than one hour since the victim ingested the poison. Do not give the victim anything to eat or drink unless told to do so. Do not rely on poisoning instructions given on container labels.

5 **Place the victim in the recovery position** *(page 13)*.

6 **Save any vomit for medical personnel.**

IMPORTANT!

- If chemicals have splashed or spilled into the victim's eyes, see Eye Emergencies *(page 28)*.

- If chemicals have splashed or spilled on to the victim's skin, see Burns *(page 15)*.

- If the victim inhaled poisonous gas, take him to fresh air and then begin the first-aid steps for poisoning described here.

- Since a poisoning victim may exhibit few symptoms or symptoms that are not listed below, it is very important to examine the scene for clues.

SYMPTOMS

- Headache
- Dizziness
- Fever
- Abdominal pain
- Vision problems
- Seizures
- Unusual breath odour
- Chills
- Drowsiness
- Burns on skin
- Nausea or vomiting
- Breathing problems
- Unconsciousness

POISONOUS SUBSTANCES

You may be surprised at the large number of potentially lethal substances in your home. To a child a mothball looks like a sweet, cough syrup and nail varnish resemble fruit drinks, and bleach could be water. The follwing table is a comprehensive list of both common and less common poisons which, if children may be around, should be kept well of reach.

Alcohol	Nail varnish
Antifreeze	Nail varnish remover
Barbiturates	Paint
Benzodiazephines	Paracetamol
Bleach	Paraquat
Carbon monoxide	Perfume
Caustic soda	Pesticides
Cough syrup	Petrol
Deadly nightshade	Phosphorus
Dry cleaning solvents	Plasticine
Foxglove	Shoe creams and polishes
Fuels	Slug pellets
Holly	Snake bites
Household drugs	Solvents
Illegal drugs	Tobacco
Insecticides	Turpentine
Iodine	Vitamins A and D
Laburnum	Weedkiller
Lead	White Spirit
Lighter fuel	Windscreen cleaner
Matches	Wood preservative treatments
Mothballs	Yew

SEIZURES

◆ If this is the first time the victim has had a seizure, if the victim has more than one seizure per hour, or if the seizure lasts more than two minutes, telephone 999.

◆ Seizures, while frightening, are usually not life-threatening. You should be more concerned about the seizure's cause, so be sure to determine if the victim is wearing a medical identi-bracelet or if he is suffering from another injury.

SYMPTOMS

◆ Tingling sensation
◆ Twitching, muscle spasms
◆ Body stiffening
◆ Drooling
◆ Loss of bladder or bowel control
◆ Temporary respiratory arrest
◆ Unconsciousness

CAUTION: If you suspect a head, neck, or back injury, see page 32.

1 **If the victim suspects that he is going to have a seizure or if he begins to lose his balance, help him to the ground.**

2 **Lay the victim on his side to prevent any vomit from entering his lungs.** CAUTION: Do not put your hands in or near the victim's mouth during the seizure.

3 **Loosen any tight clothing on the victim.**

4 **Prevent the victim from injuring himself.** Remove spectacles. Push away any objects or furniture that might injure the victim if he collides with it. CAUTION: Do not try to restrict his movements, unless he is going to hurt himself.

5 **When the seizure has ended, help the victim into a comfortable position on his side.** The victim is likely to be tired and confused; he may fall asleep.

6 **Check the victim's ABCs** *(page 13).* **If the victim is not breathing or does not have a pulse or heartbeat, begin CPR** *(pages 16-17).*

FEBRILE SEIZURES

Seizures in young children or infants are often caused by sudden high fevers. If the child has such a fever, take off his clothes and sponge his body with luke-warm, not cold, water. Call your doctor for further advice. CAUTION: Do not give the child a bath.

SHOCK

IMPORTANT!

◆ Telephone 999.

SYMPTOMS

◆ Restlessness or anxiety
◆ Weak, rapid pulse
◆ Cold, clammy, pale skin
◆ Shaking chills
◆ Chest pain
◆ Rapid, shallow breathing
◆ Dizziness or general weakness
◆ Nausea or vomiting
◆ Unconsciousness

CAUTION: If you suspect a head, neck, or back injury, see page 32.

1 Check the victim's ABCs *(page 13)*. **If the victim is not breathing or does not have a pulse or heartbeat, begin CPR** *(pages 16-17).*

2 Position the victim so he is comfortable. Unless the victim is more comfortable sitting up, lay him on his back, with his head lower than the rest of his body. If you do not suspect any broken leg bones, elevate the legs 20 to 30 centimetres. Recheck the victim's airway.

3 Try to determine the cause of shock and perform first aid for the appropriate emergency.

4 Make the victim warm and comfortable. Loosen any tight clothing and cover the victim with a blanket or additional clothing. Do not use an electric blanket or any other form of direct heat. If the victim is lying down, do not place a pillow under the head, as this might cause the airway to become blocked.

5 Keep the airway open. If the victim begins to choke or vomit, turn his head to one side so that the vomit will not block his airway.

6 If medical help is more than an hour away, give the conscious victim a clean cloth soaked in water to suck on.

ANAPHYLACTIC SHOCK

IMPORTANT!
◆ If you suspect a severe allergic reaction, the victim may be in anaphylactic shock.

SYMPTOMS
◆ Itching
◆ Flushed face
◆ Dizziness
◆ Nausea or vomiting
◆ Wheezing
◆ Unconsciousness
◆ Hives
◆ Warm skin
◆ Swollen face or tongue
◆ Abdominal cramps
◆ Difficulty in breathing

In addition to treating the victim as you would for shock, perform these steps:

◆ **Try to keep the victim calm.**

◆ **Determine if the victim was stung by an insect.** If so, carefully scrape the sting off the victim's skin. CAUTION: Do not use tweezers; this may push more venom into the skin.

◆ **Administer medicine, if available.** Some people are prone to anaphylactic shock and may have emergency supplies on hand. If this is the case, help the victim with his medicine. This may include giving the victim an injection of adrenaline; follow the instructions on the medication.

YOUR MEDICINE CHEST

CONVENTIONAL

It is helpful to have some medications for common ailments on hand in your home so that when the occasional cold or flu strikes you'll be prepared. All of the items below are available over the counter (OTC) at most chemists and supermarkets. When it comes to brand names among OTC classes, most preparations have the same active ingredients and differ only in packaging. Keep in mind that OTC products are still drugs and can have potentially dangerous side effects if misused.

All of these substances should be stored away from light, humidity, and the reach of children. Check expiration dates on all your medications periodically; many of these preparations have a limited shelf life.

Members of your family may have other, specific needs, such as adrenaline for bee allergies. These should also be included in your home medicine chest.

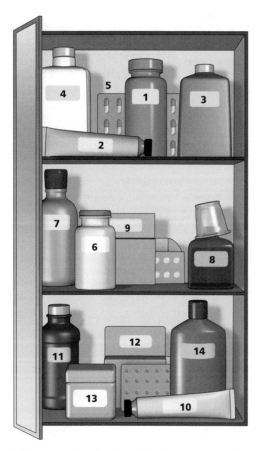

FIRST-AID SUPPLIES

In addition to your home pharmacy, you should also keep a supply of bandages and first-aid materials on hand for emergencies. These items should be stored in clean, airtight containers.

- Adhesive bandages, assorted sizes
- Adhesive tape
- Antiseptic wipes and cream
- Butterfly bandages
- Cold packs (disposable)
- Cotton, both roll and balls
- Cotton wool buds
- Elastic bandages
- Eyebath
- Gauze bandages, various sizes, in pads and rolls
- Hand mirror (to check for breathing)
- Hand wipes (disposable)
- Insect repellent
- Latex gloves
- Plasters
- Safety pins
- Scissors (kept solely for this purpose)
- Sling (triangular bandage)
- Soap
- Sterile nonstick dressings
- Thermometer (if there are children under age five in the household, be sure to include a rectal or ear thermometer or an LCD strip thermometer)
- Tissues
- Tongue depressors (for finger splints)
- Tweezers

CONVENTIONAL PRODUCTS

1 **Antacid** indigestion
2 **Antibiotic cream** cuts, scratches
3 **Antidiarrhoeal medication**
4 **Antifungal medication** athlete's foot
5 **Antihistamine capsules** and **cream** allergies and stings
6 **Aspirin** and **paracetamol** pain such as headaches or muscle cramps
7 **Calamine lotion** itching of skin rashes and insect bites
8 **Cough/cold/flu medicine** and **cough syrup**
9 **Hydrocortisone cream** skin rashes and insect bites
10 **Hydrogen peroxide** antiseptic cream for cuts and scratches
11 **Iodine**
12 **Laxative** constipation
13 **Lipsalve**
14 **Motion sickness medication**
15 **Oil of cloves**
16 **Petroleum jelly** chafing
17 **Sunscreen**
18 **Surgical spirit**

COMPLEMENTARY

Natural preparations can be used for many common ailments. These herbs, oils, and homeopathic medications can usually be found at health food stores or specialized pharmacies. Oils and homeopathic pharmaceuticals are commonly prepackaged, but herbs may be purchased loose and combined at home to create specific preparations. Don't forget that herbs, like OTC drugs, are powerful substances and should be used with care.

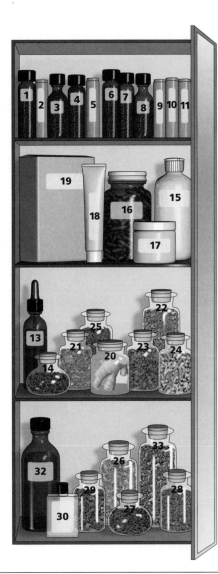

HOMEOPATHIC

1 Aconite colds, croup, fever, shock

2 Apis bites and stings, hives

3 Arnica bruises, dislocated joints, shock

4 Arsenicum album colds, food poisoning, influenza

5 Belladonna earache, fever, headache, infection, heatstroke

6 Bryonia back pain, fever, headaches, influenza

7 Calcium carbonate allergy, catarrh

8 Gelsemium fever and influenza

9 Hepar sulphuris abscesses, boils, croup, sore throat

10 Hypericum injury to nerves, insect bites

11 Nux vomica over-eating, hangover, headache, respiratory problems

12 Pulsatilla childhood infections, colds, fever, sinus problem, aches and pains

13 Rescue remedy alternative to aconite and arnica

14 Rhus toxicodendron back pain, chickenpox, influenza, sprains, strains

HERBAL

15 Aloe (*Aloe vera*) apply gel externally for bee stings, sunburn

16 Chamomile (*Chamaemelum nobile*) tea for indigestion

17 Chickweed (*Stellaria media*) cream for relief of skin irritation

18 Comfrey (*Symphytum officinale*) leaf ointment for cuts but not puncture wounds

19 Dandelion (*Taraxacum officinale*) root decoction as a secretory laxative

20 Elder (*Sambucus nigra*) flower, **peppermint** (*Mentha piperita*), and **yarrow** (*Achillea millefolium*) hot infusion of equal parts three times daily to relieve sinus pain

21 Flaxseed bulk laxative

22 Gentian (*Gentiana lutea*) hot tea to relieve indigestion

23 Ginger (*Zingiber officinale*) hot infusion of root as needed to relieve nausea

24 Marshmallow (*Althaea officinalis*) hot infusion as needed for coughs

25 Meadowsweet (*Filipendula ulmaria*), **American cranesbill** (*Geranium maculatum*), and **peppermint** (*Mentha piperita*) infusion of equal parts to relieve symptoms of diarrhoea

26 Mullein (*Verbascum thapsus*) hot infusion three times daily for coughs; useful for children

27 Peppermint (*Mentha piperita*) tea or infusion to relieve indigestion, diarrhoea

28 Psyllium (*Plantago psyllium*) bulk laxative

29 Sage (*Salvia officinalis*) gargle infusion for sore throat

30 Tea tree oil (*Melaleuca alternifolia*) externally for athlete's foot

31 White horehound (*Marrubium vulgare*) hot infusion as needed for coughs

32 Witch hazel (*Hamamelis virginiana*) distilled, use externally for relief of itching

33 Yellow dock (*Rumex crispus*) decoction three times daily as secretory laxative

■

AILMENTS
AND OPTIONS ▶

ABDOMINAL PAINS

Read down this column to find your symptoms. Then read across.

SYMPTOMS	AILMENT/PROBLEM
◆ pain in the abdomen; burning feeling in the chest; chest pain, particularly after eating or drinking alcohol; wind or belching; nausea; acid taste in mouth.	◆ Acid stomach; indigestion; heartburn
◆ cramping or pain in the abdomen; nausea; diarrhoea; vomiting; fever; malaise; weakness; intestinal wind.	◆ Gastroenteritis
◆ abdominal discomfort, pain, or cramping; pain under the breastbone; possibly, nausea.	◆ Gastritis
◆ pain in the abdomen or under the breastbone, often at night or one hour after eating; pain usually relieved by eating or vomiting; possibly, black-appearing stools.	◆ Peptic ulcer
◆ pain in the abdomen accompanied by diarrhoea or constipation, especially after eating; relief with defecation.	◆ Irritable bowel syndrome
◆ cramping or pain in the abdomen; fever; loss of appetite; weight loss; diarrhoea; wind; rectal bleeding.	◆ Inflammatory bowel disease; ulcerative colitis; Crohn's disease
◆ sharp, steady pain in groin; lump in abdomen when standing or straining.	◆ Inguinal hernia
◆ intense, sudden pain in upper-right abdomen, especially after a fatty meal; pain may move to right shoulder blade, may last several hours, and is followed by general abdominal soreness. Nausea, vomiting.	◆ Gallstones

WHAT TO DO	OTHER INFO
◆ Adjust your eating and drinking habits or take an antacid to reduce the symptoms.	◆ Avoid smoking, caffeine, alcohol, eating too quickly, junk food and nonsteroidal anti-inflammatory drugs (NSAIDs), such as aspirin.
◆ Rest and drink plenty of fluids.	◆ Gastroenteritis is inflammation of the stomach or intestines often caused by a virus or food poisoning. Hospitalization may be required if symptoms are severe or the patient is very young, elderly, or debilitated.
◆ Take only liquids for one day; then reintroduce solid food into the diet in small amounts.	◆ Gastritis, an inflammation of the stomach lining, may be caused by lifestyle factors, such as heavy drinking, smoking, or overeating; using aspirin, ibuprofen, or prescription drugs; or a bacterial infection.
◆ Rest; eat small, frequent meals; take antacids; avoid smoking, alcohol, aspirin, and caffeine. Your doctor may prescribe a histamine H_2 blocker. If stools appear black, the ulcer may be bleeding. **Call your doctor now.**	◆ If the symptoms persist or recur, your doctor will want to test you for the presence of *Helicobacter pylori*, the bacterium known to be the leading cause of peptic ulcers. Treatment is with antibiotics.
◆ The usual first step for reducing symptoms is to take a fibre-based laxative or an antidiarrhoeal drug.	◆ Adding fibre and fluid to the diet is important, as is exercise. Because stress appears to be a trigger, counselling, biofeedback, yoga, or meditation may be helpful.
◆ **Call your doctor now.** A medical evaluation is necessary for diagnosis and treatment.	◆ Various alternative therapies, such as drinking green leafy vegetable juices for the chlorophyll content, may relieve symptoms. In severe cases, surgery is required to remove all or part of the damaged intestine.
◆ **Call your doctor now.**	◆ In this disorder, the intestines or bladder bulges through the abdominal wall.
◆ **Call your doctor now**. A medical evaluation is necessary for diagnosis and treatment, which may involve surgical removal of the gallbladder or a nonsurgical procedure that dissolves the stones.	◆ Reducing fat and meat intake and increasing fibre may help prevent the formation of new stones.

SYMPTOMS	AILMENT/PROBLEM
◆ acute, constant abdominal pain radiating to the back and chest; fever; nausea; vomiting; abdominal distention; clammy skin.	◆ Pancreatitis
◆ severe cramping pain that is usually worse on the left side of the abdomen; chills; fever; nausea; history of constipation.	◆ Diverticulitis
◆ sharp pain in the side that moves toward the groin and/or abdomen; frequent urge to urinate; blocked flow of urine; painful urination; cloudy or foul-smelling urine; blood in urine; fever and chills; nausea and vomiting; profuse sweating.	◆ Kidney stones
◆ pain low in the abdomen that is accompanied by painful and frequent urination; constant urge to urinate; possibly, blood in urine.	◆ Urinary tract infection
◆ pain radiating from below the breastbone into the neck and arms; heartburn; vomiting; belching; bloating; difficulty swallowing.	◆ Hiatal hernia
◆ crampy pain in the pelvic area during menstruation.	◆ Menstrual cramps
◆ extremely severe abdominal pain with or without other acute symptoms.	◆ **Emergency conditions:** intestinal obstruction, peritonitis, appendicitis, ileus, pelvic inflammatory disease, heart attack, abdominal aortic aneurysm, ischemic bowel, ruptured ectopic pregnancy, ruptured ovarian cyst, perforated peptic ulcer, anaphylactic shock, chemical burn, diabetic emergency, poisoning.

WHAT TO DO	OTHER INFO
◆ **Call your doctor now** to avoid possible life-threatening complications.	◆ The cause is usually heavy drinking or gall-bladder disease. To control chronic pancreatitis, avoid alcohol and fatty foods.
◆ **Call your doctor now.** Severe cases may require hospitalization and surgery. Treatment for milder cases usually involves bed rest, stool softeners, a liquid diet, antibiotics, and possibly, antispasmodic drugs.	◆ Although you should eat low-bulk foods during the inflammatory period, a high-fibre diet may be preventive.
◆ **Call your doctor now.** A medical evaluation is necessary for diagnosis and treatment. Commonly, the first step is to drink plenty of water and take a pain reliever until the stone passes.	◆ Infection, blockage, or large stones may make surgery necessary. A new treatment method uses high-energy shock waves to break up the stones without surgery.
◆ If you also have fever, chills, back pain, and possibly, nausea and vomiting, you may have a kidney infection. **Call your doctor now.** See Bladder Infections.	◆ Pregnant women, people with diabetes, and nursing-home patients are at greatest risk for serious complications of a urinary tract infection.
◆ **Call your doctor now.**	◆ Lifestyle changes that may alleviate symptoms include avoiding smoking and alcohol, eating smaller meals and none within two hours of going to bed.
◆ Take a pain reliever such as aspirin or ibuprofen.	◆ Chiropractic, acupuncture, or magnesium supplements may help. For severe cramps, your doctor may recommend a prescription anti-inflammatory drug.
◆ **Call your doctor or 999 now. Follow instructions to obtain immediate medical care.**	

SYMPTOMS

- Sneezing, wheezing, nasal congestion, and coughing indicate asthma, or drug or respiratory allergies.
- Itchy eyes, mouth, and throat are symptoms of respiratory allergies.
- Stomachache, frequent indigestion, and heartburn are signs of food sensitivities.
- Irritated, itchy, reddening, or swelling skin is associated with drug, food, and insect sting allergies.
- Stiffness, pain, and swelling of joints may indicate food or drug allergies.

CALL YOUR DOCTOR IF:

- you have violent stomach cramps, vomiting, bloating, or diarrhea; this could point to a serious food or other allergic reaction or food poisoning.
- breathing becomes extremely difficult or painful; you may be experiencing an asthma episode, another serious allergic reaction, or a heart attack. **Get emergency medical treatment: telephone 999.**
- you suddenly develop skin welts, accompanied by intense flushing and itching; your heart may also be beating rapidly. These symptoms may indicate the onset of anaphylactic shock, an extremely serious allergic reaction. **Get emergency medical treatment: telephone 999.** *(See also Shock in Emergencies/First Aid.)*

The term *allergy* applies to an abnormal reaction by your immune system to a substance that is usually not harmful. Allergies come in a variety of forms and vary in severity from mildly bothersome to life-threatening. An estimated one-fifth of the western hemisphere's population suffers from allergies. No one knows why some people develop them, but heredity seems to play a role in their development. Although allergies may flare up and subside throughout your life, people rarely acquire new ones past the age of 40.

The immune system protects the body from foreign substances—known as antigens—by producing antibodies and other chemicals to fight against them. Usually, the immune system ignores benign substances, such as food, and fights only dangerous ones, such as bacteria. A person develops an allergic reaction when the immune system cannot tell the good from the bad and releases a type of chemical called histamine to attack the harmless substance as if it were a threat. Histamine produces many of the symptoms associated with allergies. Substances that may trigger allergic reactions, known as allergens, range from pollen to pet dander to penicillin.

Most allergic reactions are not serious, but some, such as anaphylaxis, can be fatal *(box, page 50)*. Only a few allergies can be cured outright, but a variety of conventional and complementary treatments are available to relieve the symptoms. If your allergy is severe, it is vital that you visit a conventional medical doctor and get immediate treatment on an emergency basis.

CAUSES

Allergies come in many distinct forms and are typically grouped in general categories according to the types of substances that cause them or the parts of the body they affect.

Skin allergies: Contact dermatitis is caused by direct, topical exposure to a specific allergen; atopic dermatitis has no known cause, but it is usually hereditary. Hives, or urticaria, is an eruption of itchy, swollen, reddened welts that can last for minutes or days. Angioedema (a variant of urticaria) is characterized by a deeper swelling around the eyes and lips, and sometimes of the hands and feet as well. Both hives and angioedema stem from the body's adverse reaction to certain foods, pollen, animal dander, drugs, insect stings, cold, heat, light, or even emotional stress.

Respiratory allergies: Typical symptoms of hay fever (allergic rhinitis) include itchy eyes, nose, and roof of mouth or throat, along with nasal congestion, coughing, and sneezing. If you (or members of your family) have other allergies such as dermatitis or asthma, you are more likely to have hay fever. The terms *allergic rhinitis* and *hay fever* apply specifically to reactions caused by the pollens of grasses and other plants whose pollen is spread by the wind. But the same symptoms can be produced by other airborne substances that you inhale. These can include moulds, dust, and animal dander. If, for example, you are allergic to pet dander (dead skin scales and saliva), being near a cat will make you sneeze, wheeze, and sniffle. Mould allergies are caused by airborne spores. Outdoor moulds thrive in warm seasons or climates, while indoor moulds grow year round in damp locations (basements and bathrooms, for example). Dust causes allergies because it harbours offenders such as pollen, mould spores, and microscopic dust mites; it may also contain irritating fibres from fabrics, upholstery, and carpets.

Asthma: Asthma has various causes, but the chief ones are allergies to pollen, mould spores, animal dander, and dust mites.

Food allergies: An estimated 70 per cent of people with food allergies are under 30; most are children under the age of 6. It is sometimes difficult to pinpoint the specific allergens responsible for a food allergy, because reactions are often delayed or may be caused by food additives or even by eating habits. However, approximately 90 per cent of food allergies are caused by proteins in cow's milk, egg whites, peanuts, wheat, or soybeans. Other common food allergens include berries, shellfish, corn, beans, yellow food dye, and gum arabic (an additive in processed foods). The classic symptoms of food allergies include stomach cramps, diarrhoea, and nausea. In more severe cases, there may be vomiting, swelling of the face and tongue, and respiratory congestion, as well as dizziness, sweating, and faintness.

Drug allergies: The most common drug allergy is to drugs in the penicillin family. Other common drug allergens include sulphas, barbiturates, anticonvulsants, insulin, local anesthetics, and dyes injected into blood vessels for x-rays. Many people have reactions to aspirin; these responses are not true allergies but rather 'sensitivities.'

Insect sting allergies: Some studies speculate that people who have other allergies (food, drug, or respiratory) may be more susceptible to insect sting allergies, which affect about 15 per cent of the population. Venom in stings of bees and wasps is a common allergen.

FOOD ALLERGY OR INTOLERANCE?

More than one out of five Britons believe that they are allergic to certain foods, but fewer than 1 per cent have genuine allergies; most are unable to tolerate certain foods, often because they lack an enzyme needed for proper digestion.

Some people are sensitive to lactose, a sugar found in milk; in general, however, they can tolerate dairy products such as yogurt, sour cream, and hard cheese. Some children cannot tolerate gluten, found in wheat products. Monosodium glutamate (MSG), a flavour enhancer, can cause flushing, headaches, and numbness. Some preservatives and colourings, used in foods and wines, can cause sensitivity as well as trigger allergic reactions.

DIAGNOSTIC AND TEST PROCEDURES

After taking a full family and personal medical history, your physician will ask you a series of questions about your exposure and reactions to various allergens to eliminate and identify your allergies' causes. You may be asked to keep track of potential allergens and your allergic reactions for a week to aid in diagnosis. After this, your physician will choose a testing method.

The most common test for respiratory, penicillin, insect sting, skin, and food allergies is a skin test. A small amount of the allergen is placed on, or injected just underneath, the skin, and the physician watches for allergic symptoms. The symptoms—swelling, itchiness, and redness—generally appear within 20 minutes. Skin tests are not completely reliable, because if too much of the allergen is administered, even a nonallergic person may react. Also, extremely sensitive people may go into anaphylactic shock from skin tests. An alternative for respiratory allergies is RAST (for radioallergosorbent test), which measures the levels in the bloodstream of the antibodies associated with allergies.

TREATMENT

The best treatment for allergies is to avoid the substances that trigger them, but this can be difficult. The basic medications for allergies are antihistamines, which counteract the histamine chemicals that cause the allergic reactions. Prescription corticosteroid drugs may also be used for severe symptoms. In emergency situations—when anaphylactic shock occurs—injections of adrenaline are used to dilate bronchial passages. Immunotherapy, or allergy injections, may cure some allergies by introducing small amounts of the offending allergens in order to help the body learn to deal with them.

CONVENTIONAL MEDICINE

Skin allergies: Atopic and contact dermatitis can be treated with a variety of corticosteroids, usually hydrocortisone. Hives and angioedema often

WHAT TRIGGERS ANAPHYLACTIC SHOCK?

The most severe and dangerous of allergic reactions is anaphylaxis, or anaphylactic shock, which begins within minutes after exposure and advances quickly. Although any allergen can trigger anaphylactic shock, the most common are insect stings, certain foods (such as shellfish and nuts), and injections of certain drugs. Standard emergency treatment includes an injection of epinephrine to open up the airways and blood vessels; in severe cases, cardiopulmonary resuscitation (CPR) may be necessary. See Shock in Emergencies/First Aid.

need no medication, but severe cases may require prescription antihistamines, cimetidine, terbutaline, or oral corticosteroids.

Respiratory allergies: Hay fever is generally treated with over-the-counter antihistamines, but your doctor may prescribe other, more powerful drugs—such as sodium cromoglycate—if your symptoms are severe. The same treatments apply to other respiratory allergies, but if your symptoms are severe, your physician may prescribe corticosteroids, in nasal spray or oral form. Immunotherapy has a high success rate, curing 70 per cent to 80 per cent of people treated for respiratory allergies.

Food allergies: The best treatment for food allergies is avoidance. If your reactions to certain foods are irritating but not life-endangering, your doctor may prescribe antihistamines or topical creams to help relieve symptoms.

Drug allergies: The only effective treatment for drug allergies is avoidance. Skin rashes associated with drug allergies are generally treated with antihistamines; occasionally, they are treated with corticosteroids.

Insect sting allergies: Avoidance is the best treatment, but immunotherapy may cure insect sting allergies. If you are extremely allergic and likely to go into anaphylactic shock, your doctor will prescribe an emergency kit, which you must carry with you at all times.

COMPLEMENTARY CHOICES

Since allergies can be difficult to diagnose, and are often incurable, complementary remedies for them have become quite popular. But if you have a severe allergy, or in case of an emergency, you must see a conventional physician.

ACUPRESSURE

To relieve symptoms associated with respiratory allergies, try Large Intestine 4, the highest spot of the area between the index finger and thumb; rub firmly for one minute, then repeat on the other hand. Do not use this point if you are pregnant. To fortify the immune system, firmly massage Triple Warmer 5, two finger widths from your wrist on the top of your forearm, specifically the area between the two arm bones.

AROMATHERAPY

To relieve nasal congestion, try mixing 1 drop of lavender *(Lavandula officinalis)* oil and 1 tsp of a carrier oil such as sweet almond or sunflower oil; massage into the skin around your sinuses once a day. Eucalyptus *(Eucalyptus globulus)*, cedarwood, and peppermint *(Mentha piperita)* oils also act as decongestants; dab on a handkerchief and inhale.

CHINESE HERBS

Ephedra *(Ephedra sinica)* acts like the decongestant adrenaline, which opens up the lungs' airways when breathing is difficult. But be careful: Large quantities of this herb are equivalent to large quantities of the drug adrenaline and can have serious side effects. Do not use ephedra if you have high blood pressure or heart disease. Prepare an infusion by combining 5 grams ephedra, 4 grams cinnamon *(Cinnamomum cassia)* sticks, 1.5 grams licorice *(Glycyrrhiza glabra)*, and 5 grams apricot seed *(Prunus armeniaca)*; let steep in cold water, then bring to a boil. Strain and drink hot.

HERBAL THERAPIES

Infusions of chamomile *(Chamaemelum nobile)*, elder *(Sambucus nigra)* flower, eyebright *(Euphrasia rostkoviana)*, garlic *(Allium sativum)*, goldenrod *(Solidago virgaurea)*, nettle *(Urtica dioica)*, and yarrow *(Achillea millefolium)* have antimucus and anti-inflammatory effects.

HOMEOPATHY

For a runny nose, itchy throat, and sneezing, a homeopathic practitioner might suggest Arsenicum album (6c); for chronic thick mucus, Pulsatilla (6c); for a runny nose, sore upper lip, and itchy eyes, Allium cepa (6c).

NUTRITION AND DIET

Vitamin C and bioflavonoids (found in the white pith of citrus fruits) act as natural antihistamines, so you should increase your citrus intake or take 500 mg of vitamin C three times daily. Vitamins A and B complex are thought to be stimulants to the immune system. Products made with bee pollen and royal jelly may alleviate or eliminate the symptoms of respiratory allergies but should not be taken if you are allergic to bee stings. For food allergies, read labels carefully and make sure you know which foods to avoid.

PREVENTION

Respiratory allergies: Install a high-efficiency air cleaner to help remove pollen and mould spores, and use an air conditioner in your home and car during warm seasons to keep pollen out; regularly clean damp areas with bleach to kill moulds. Consider hiring a specialist cleaning service to rid furniture and upholstery of dust mites. Isolate (or, if you can stand it, get rid of) your pets and keep them outside as much as possible. Regular baths for your pet will help reduce dander.

Food allergies: Instead of dairy products, try tofu-based foods. Always check food labels for additives that are known allergens, such as yellow food dye and gum arabic. ■

SYMPTOMS

- Pain and progressive stiffness without noticeable swelling, chills, or fever during normal activities probably indicate the gradual onset of **osteoarthritis.**
- Painful swelling, inflammation, and stiffness in the arms, legs, wrists, or fingers in the same joints on both sides of the body, especially on awakening, may be signs of **rheumatoid arthritis.**
- Fever, joint inflammation, tenderness, and sharp pain, sometimes accompanied by chills and associated with an injury or another illness, may indicate **infectious arthritis.**
- In children, intermittent fever, loss of appetite, weight loss, anaemia, or blotchy rash on the arms and legs may signal **juvenile rheumatoid arthritis.**

CALL YOUR DOCTOR IF:

- the pain and stiffness come on quickly, whether from an injury or an unknown cause; you may be experiencing the onset of **rheumatoid arthritis.**
- the pain is accompanied by fever; you may have **infectious arthritis.**
- you notice pain and stiffness in your arms, legs, or back after sitting for short periods or after a night's sleep; you may be developing **osteoarthritis** or another arthritic condition.
- a child develops pain or a rash on armpits, knees, wrists, and ankles, or has fever swings, poor appetite, and weight loss; the child may have **juvenile rheumatoid arthritis.**

The British workforce loses more time to pain in the joints than to any other type of ailment. To the extent that our jobs and leisure activities become more sedentary, the likelihood of such ailments increases. Fortunately, many of the problems commonly labelled 'arthritis' are easily healed or controlled, and the prospects of debilitating complications are far less than they were for our parents and grandparents.

Although the term is applied to a wide variety of disorders, arthritis means the inflammation of a joint, whether as the result of a disease, an infection, a genetic defect, or some other cause. Many people, however, perceive it as any kind of pain or discomfort associated with body movement, including such localized problems as low back pain, bursitis, tendonitis, and general stiffness or pain in the joints. *(See also Backache.)*

For many—although by no means everyone—arthritis seems to be an inevitable part of the aging process, and there are no signs of real cures on the immediate horizon. On the positive side, advances in both conventional medical treatment and complementary therapies make living with arthritis more bearable.

MAJOR TYPES OF ARTHRITIS

Rheumatoid arthritis, sometimes called rheumatism or synovitis, tends to affect people over the age of 40, and women two to three times as commonly as men. It may occur in children, particularly girls from 2 to 5 years of age. It is characterized by inflammation and pain in the hands—especially the knuckles and second joints—as well as in the arms, legs, and feet, and by general fatigue and sleeplessness. It can also cause systemic damage to other parts of the body, including the heart, lungs, eyes, nerves, and muscles. The discomfort of rheumatoid arthritis can develop over weeks or months and tends to be most severe on awakening.

Rheumatoid arthritis in older people may eventually cause the hands and feet to become gnarled and misshapen as muscles weaken, tendons shrink, and the ends of bones become abnormally enlarged.

While there is no complete cure, treatment

begun at the onset of the disorder relieves symptoms in most people. Symptoms may endure for five years or more, after which they tend to stabilize or decline. With early treatment, the likelihood of permanent disability is reduced in all but 5 to 10 per cent of sufferers.

Juvenile rheumatoid arthritis, or Still's disease, is characterized by chronic fever and anaemia. The disease can also have secondary effects on the heart, lungs, eyes, and nervous system. Arthritic episodes in children younger than the age of five can last for several weeks and may recur, although the symptoms tend to be less severe in recurrent attacks. Treatment is essentially the same as for adults, with heavy emphasis on physical therapy and exercise to keep growing bodies active. Permanent damage from juvenile rheumatoid arthritis is now rare, and most affected children recover from the disease fully without experiencing any lasting disabilities.

Infectious arthritis refers to various ailments that affect larger arm and leg joints as well as the fingers or toes. Arthritic infection is usually a complication of an injury or of another disease and is much less common than arthritic conditions that come on with age. Because the symptoms may be masked by the primary injury or illness, however, infectious arthritis may go unnoticed and, if left untreated, can result in permanent disability.

Osteoarthritis, or degenerative joint disease, refers to the pain and inflammation that can result from the systematic loss of bone tissue in the joints. It is the most common form of arthritis, particularly in the elderly. In osteoarthritis, the protective cartilage at the ends of bones in joints—especially in the spine and legs—gradually wears away. The inner bone surfaces become exposed and rub together. In some cases, bony spurs develop on the edges of joints, causing damage to muscles and nerves, pain, deformity, and difficulty in movement.

Although the mechanism of osteoarthritis is unknown, some people appear to have a genetic predisposition to degenerative bone disorders. In rare cases, congenital bone deformation appears at an early age. Misuse of anabolic steroids, which are popular among some athletes, can also bring on early osteoarthritic degeneration.

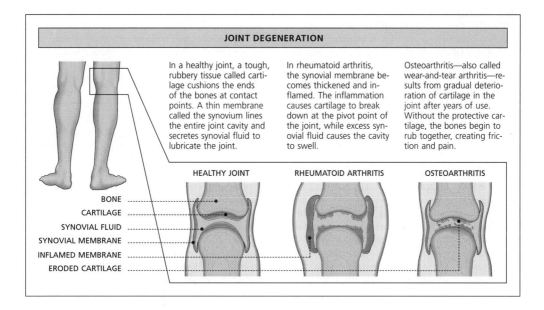

JOINT DEGENERATION

In a healthy joint, a tough, rubbery tissue called cartilage cushions the ends of the bones at contact points. A thin membrane called the synovium lines the entire joint cavity and secretes synovial fluid to lubricate the joint.

In rheumatoid arthritis, the synovial membrane becomes thickened and inflamed. The inflammation causes cartilage to break down at the pivot point of the joint, while excess synovial fluid causes the cavity to swell.

Osteoarthritis—also called wear-and-tear arthritis—results from gradual deterioration of cartilage in the joint after years of use. Without the protective cartilage, the bones begin to rub together, creating friction and pain.

HEALTHY JOINT   RHEUMATOID ARTHRITIS   OSTEOARTHRITIS

BONE
CARTILAGE
SYNOVIAL FLUID
SYNOVIAL MEMBRANE
INFLAMED MEMBRANE
ERODED CARTILAGE

In many people the onset of osteoarthritis is gradual and has no serious debilitating effect, although it can change the shape and size of bones. In other people, bony growths and gnarled joints may cause painful muscle inflammation or nerve damage, along with significant changes in posture and mobility.

Other arthritic conditions include ankylosing spondylitis (arthritis of the spine), bone spurs (bony growths on the vertebrae or other areas), gout, and systemic lupus (inflammatory connective-tissue disease).

CAUSES

Each of the three major types of arthritic condition has its own apparent causes:

Rheumatoid arthritis. The cause of rheumatoid arthritis is not fully understood. Some researchers think it may be some sort of autoimmune disorder. Another theory suggests that it is an immune reaction to a viral infection in the body.

Infectious arthritis. This type of arthritis is caused by a bacterial or viral invasion of the joints and typically comes on the heels of another disease, such as staphylococcus infection, tuberculosis, gonorrhoea, or Lyme disease.

Osteoarthritis. This common degenerative joint disease is part of the ageing process. The condition may be associated with broken bones and can develop in young adults from wear and tear on the body's load-bearing joints, often as a result of intense athletic activity. In cases of osteoarthritis, the cartilage and bone cannot repair themselves sufficiently to keep up with the damage.

DIAGNOSTIC AND TEST PROCEDURES
In addition to symptom analysis, blood tests are commonly used to confirm **rheumatoid arthritis;** the majority of sufferers have antibodies called rheumatoid factors (RF) in their blood, although RF may also be present in other disorders.

X-rays are used to diagnose **osteoarthritis,** typically revealing shrunken joints or calcification at the ends of the bones. If your doctor suspects **in-fectious arthritis** as a complication of some other disease, testing a sample of fluid from the affected joint will usually confirm the diagnosis.

TREATMENT

Sometimes arthritic damage can be slowed or stopped, but in most cases the damage continues as the disease runs its course, regardless of whether drugs or other therapies are used to relieve the symptoms. Predictably, the duration and intensity of the actual pain and discomfort depend on the type of arthritis and the degree of severity. The process may take a few days in the case of minor joint problems in otherwise healthy adults, while in others it may last months or years. In older people with severe rheumatoid or degenerative conditions, for example, the effects may be lifelong.

CONVENTIONAL MEDICINE
In the case of localized pain, stiffness, and immobility, the typical three-stage therapy consists of medication to relieve pain and inflammation, rest to let injured tissues heal themselves, and exercise to rebuild mobility and strength.

To reduce pain and inflammation in mild cases of **rheumatoid arthritis** and **osteoarthritis,** your doctor will probably prescribe aspirin or another nonsteroidal anti-inflammatory drug (NSAID) such as ibuprofen. Physicians may combine these drugs with regimens of heat, rest and exercise, physical therapy, and physical aids such as a walking stick or frame. Controlled application of deep heat and ultrasound can also soothe affected joints.

In more advanced cases, your doctor may recommend corticosteroid injections to ease the pain and stiffness of affected joints. Depending on the individual, results range from temporary relief to long-lasting suppression of symptoms.

Early this century, researchers discovered that certain compounds containing gold, delivered orally or by injection, gave relief to some patients and total remission in others. Note, however, that because the side effects of gold therapy can range from minor skin rash to severe blood and kidney disorders, this therapy should be approached with caution.

In cases of arthritic complications from injury or infection, specific therapy will depend on the nature and seriousness of the underlying condition. The major concern is for healing the affected area before more serious complications occur. Treatment of **infectious arthritis** typically involves large intravenous doses of antibiotics as well as drainage of excess fluid from the joints.

Various forms of surgery may be needed to reduce the discomfort of arthritis or to restore mobility. Synovectomy is the removal of damaged connective tissue lining a joint cavity, and allows the body to regenerate new, healthy tissue in its place. This operation is most common in the knee. In cases of severe arthritic damage to the neck or foot, bones can be surgically removed or fused. Although movement is limited after such surgery, the operations relieve excruciating pain and help prevent further damage to nerves or blood vessels.

If arthritic pain and inflammation become truly unbearable, or arthritic joints simply refuse to function, the answer may lie in surgical replacement. Today, hip and shoulder joints—as well as smaller joints in elbows, knees, and fingers—can be replaced with reliable artificial joints made of stainless steel and plastic.

Because one of the most trying aspects of arthritis is learning to live with pain, many doctors recommend training in pain management, including cognitive therapy. Such programmes focus on improving patients' emotional and psychological well-being by teaching them how to relax and conduct their daily activities at a realistic pace. Learning to overcome mental stress and anxiety can be the key to coping with the physical limitations that may accompany chronic rheumatoid arthritis and osteoarthritis. Cognitive therapy may include various techniques for activity scheduling, imaging, relaxation, distraction, and creative problem solving.

COMPLEMENTARY CHOICES

Because medical science has not found any full cures for the various kinds of arthritis, many people turn to alternative treatments to ease their pain and disability. While few alternative approaches can definitively be substantiated in controlled studies of their effectiveness, research indicates that some of these methods can play a significant role in treating arthritic ailments. **Meditation,** self-hypnosis, **guided imagery,** and **relaxation** techniques, for example, can have positive effects in controlling chronic arthritis pain. Arthritis sufferers should be extremely cautious,

W A R N I N G !

BEWARE OF QUACK CURES

Because neither conventional nor alternative medicine can cure rheumatoid arthritis or osteoarthritis, unproven treatments abound. Over the years, arthritis sufferers have reported relief with remedies ranging from copper bracelets to laser treatments. While such therapies claim success in individual cases, you should exercise caution and a degree of scepticism when considering what's right for you.

In general, untested and unproven remedies that aren't injected or swallowed will probably do no harm. Invasive treatments may have dangerous side effects or cause other systemic problems, however. The results, if any, may not justify the money spent. The Arthritis Foundation estimates that people from every income bracket and education level spend a fortune every year on unproven arthritis treatments.

Your best defence against unscrupulous practices is to know as much as you can about your ailment and the risks and intended benefits of suggested treatments. Understanding the underlying causes of the disease and maintaining a healthy scepticism about claims for quick cures will help you avoid placing your health and your wallet at risk.

however, about practices that claim to 'cure' the disease. Furthermore, what appears to work for one person under a given set of circumstances may not work at all for someone else.

ACUPRESSURE AND ACUPUNCTURE

Some arthritis patients find that these therapies, administered by a trained practitioner, offer effective relief from the pain of **rheumatoid arthritis** or **osteoarthritis** for several weeks or months.

BODY WORK

In combination with other treatments, soft-tissue massage around affected joints or compassionate touching by a physician or other practitioner can have a comforting, reassuring effect on those who suffer from arthritis. Manipulation by a trained therapist constitutes passive exercise for people unable to perform vigorous exercise. In addition to making a patient feel better physically, sympathetically administered touch therapy can help soothe the emotional effects of chronic illness. Studies suggest that relieving stress and tension has a positive influence on the body's hormonal balance and resistance to pain.

CHIROPRACTIC OR OSTEOPATHY

After diagnostic examination, testing, and appropriate conventional therapy, a chiropractor may manipulate the spine and other arthritic joints to relieve pain and help re-establish normal use.

HERBAL THERAPIES

Among the various remedies herbalists recommend to relieve pain is a 5-ml tincture made from 2 parts willow (*Salix* spp.) bark and 1 part each of black cohosh (*Cimicifuga racemosa*) and nettle (*Urtica dioica*), taken three times a day. To relieve muscle tension, rub a tincture of lobelia (*Lobelia inflata*) and cramp bark (*Viburnum opulus*) on the affected area.

HOMEOPATHY

For chronic **osteoarthritis** and **rheumatoid arthritis**, constitutional remedies will be prescribed after consultation with a trained homeopathic practitioner. Homeopathic remedies to relieve

---

YOGA TECHNIQUES

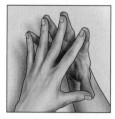 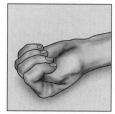

1 To loosen the joints of the hand, use the **Spider Push-Up.** Press your fingertips together firmly, palms 5 to 8 centimetres apart. Push your palms toward each other while keeping your fingertips touching. Do this 20 times.

2 To ease stiff finger joints, do the **Thumb Squeezer.** Curl your fingers into a fist around your thumb, gently squeeze, then slowly release. Do this 10 times with each hand.

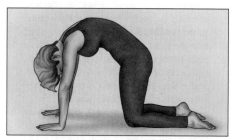

3 The Dog and **Cat** help stretch your hips and back. On your hands and knees in the table position, inhale as you lower your back and lift your head and buttocks (Dog). Then exhale as you arch your back and drop your head and buttocks (Cat). Repeat 9 times.

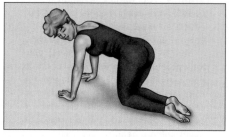

4 Do the **C** exercise on your hands and knees. Exhale and swing your head and buttocks as far to the left as you can. Breathe deeply as you hold this position for 10 seconds; exhale as you slowly straighten your back. Repeat to the right. Do this 10 times.

immediate pain and joint stiffness may include Rhus toxicodendron or Bryonia.

HYDROTHERAPY
Swimming or other water exercise, preferably in a heated pool, allows arthritis patients to work on movement of affected joints and improve muscle strength; the water helps support the body and reduce the stress of gravity.

NUTRITION AND DIET
Avoiding specific foods can stop arthritic symptoms tied to allergies, especially to grains, nuts, meats, eggs, and dairy products. Use trial and error, preferably under the supervision of an allergy specialist.

Some practitioners recommend cutting out plants in the nightshade family: tomato, potato, eggplant, and pepper. They believe the alkaloids in these foods inhibit formation of the collagen that makes up cartilage.

Low-fat, low-protein vegetarian diets may ease the pain and inflammation of **rheumatoid arthritis.** Positive results are reported from elim-

inating partially hydrogenated fats and polyunsaturated vegetable oils, and supplementing the diet with flax oil, sardines, and other oily fish as a source of omega-3 fatty acids.

Vitamin therapy may relieve certain arthritic symptoms. Beta carotene (vitamin A) has an antioxidant effect on cells, neutralizing destructive molecules called free radicals. Vitamins C, B_6, and E, as well as zinc, are thought to enhance collagen production and the repair of connective tissue. Vitamin C may also be advised for people taking aspirin, which depletes the body's vitamin C balance. Niacin (vitamin B_3) may also be helpful, although excessive use may aggravate liver problems. Always take vitamin supplements under professional guidance, since overdoses of some vitamin compounds can have side effects or undesirable interactions with drugs.

Some therapists recommend cherries or dark red berries to stimulate the production of collagen, essential to cartilage repair.

YOGA
A number of yoga positions *(opposite)* may have beneficial effects on arthritis.

HOME REMEDIES
Heat and rest—traditional remedies for arthritic pain—are very effective in the short term for most people with the disease. Overweight sufferers should begin weight reduction, especially when arthritis strikes the lower back and legs.

If arthritic pain comes on unexpectedly, supplement an over-the-counter painkiller with dry heat from a heating pad or moist heat in the form of a hot bath or a hot-water bottle wrapped in a towel. Regular exercise is important to keep the joints mobile. People with weakened, badly deformed fingers from **rheumatoid arthritis** benefit from specially designed utensils and door and drawer handles; people suffering weakness in the legs and arms from **osteoarthritis** can use special bathroom fixtures, especially bath rails and elevated toilet seats. ■

SYMPTOMS

- Pain, discomfort, restricted movement, tenderness, and possible swelling may be indicative of some form of muscle or ligament injury, such as a sprain or strain.
- Pain, swelling, tenderness, and deformity may indicate a **fracture.**
- Pain, restricted movement, misshapen appearance, and swelling in a joint are symptoms of a **dislocation.**
- Localized pain just below the kneecap may be a sign of patellar tendonitis. In adolescents, the condition may indicate Osgood-Schlatter disease if accompanied by swelling (see page 62).
- Pain in the elbow, often accompanied by tenderness in the inner or outer portion of the elbow and forearm, and possibly a weak and painful grasp, may indicate **epicondylitis.**

CALL YOUR DOCTOR IF:

- your muscles gradually become weak for no apparent reason; you may have a neurological problem or another disorder of immediate concern.
- you experience chronic muscle cramps. Although most often benign, this may be a sign of serious problems such as blood clotting, restricted blood flow, or nerve damage.
- you think your swelling or puffiness is caused by a fracture, dislocation, ligament or muscle tear, or cartilage damage. If not treated by a physician swiftly, the affected area could suffer permanent damage.

Every family has seen its share of injuries tracing to athletic activities or, ironically, the pursuit of physical fitness. For the most part, athletic injuries are a result of stress put on bones or muscles. Most common are injuries to soft tissue—muscles, tendons, and ligaments.

A **dislocation** occurs when two bones are jolted apart at a joint and is often accompanied by a ligament tear in the joint. The pain is caused by the severe stretching of soft tissues.

A **fracture** is either simple (closed)—in which the broken bone remains beneath the skin surface and does minimal damage to surrounding tissues—or compound (open)—in which the bone protrudes through the skin. The ankle, hand, wrist, and collarbone are common sites of fracture.

Shoulder injuries are common in sports that require throwing motions or intense contact. Dislocations are most common in the shoulder joint. **Acromioclavicular joint (AC) separation** occurs when the ligaments that support the collarbone are torn. The rotator cuff is where four muscles meet and attach to the humerus; overuse of the shoulder may inflame or tear tendons in the area, causing **rotator cuff tendonitis.**

CHILD SPORTS INJURIES: WHAT PARENTS SHOULD KNOW

- *Each year during the football season there are hundreds of thousands of injuries; rugby also carries a high risk of injury.*
- *Children are at a higher risk of injury than adult athletes because those playing together may be at vastly different weights, stages of development and strengths, and they are fearless. Try to ensure that participants in a group are at a similar level of physical development.*

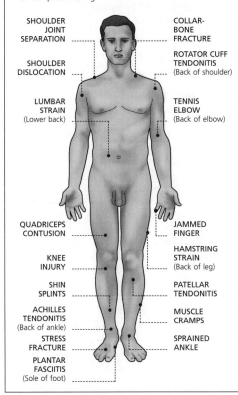

Epicondylitis affects the elbow and typically occurs in sports requiring frequent wrist manipulation and forearm rotation. The lateral (affecting the outer elbow) form is tennis elbow. Medial epicondylitis involves the inner elbow.

Lower-back injuries, such as muscle tears, are common in sports that involve a lot of bend-ing. The high velocity and full contact nature of hockey, lacrosse and football frequently cause neck and spine injuries, such as a **herniated disk,** in which an intervertebral disc protrudes from the spinal column.

Intense leg movement, including twisting and spreading, may tear the adductor muscle **(groin strain),** which connects the leg with the pubic bone.

The knees are involved in some of the most common lower-body injuries. Continual jumping may result in tearing of the tendon just below the kneecap, or patella, causing **patellar tendonitis,** or jumper's knee. The knees may also suffer from other injuries, such as tears of the meniscus, a piece of cartilage in the knee joint between the femur and tibia.

Sudden tearing of muscle fibres may occur after excessive athletic activity and the conse-quent accumulation of fluid in the muscle causes pain, tenderness, local swelling and **cramp.**

Increased interest in jogging and cross train-ing has resulted in a parallel rise in leg injuries, including shin splints, tendonitis, and **stress frac-tures,** especially in the tibia or fibula bones. If continually exposed to stress from prolonged standing, running, or walking, a stress fracture may result in a larger fracture.

The foot often falls victim to injury because it must support the weight of the entire body. **Plantar fasciitis** often affects inexperienced run-ners, causing pain along the inner heel and along the arch of the foot, sometimes accompanied by stiffness and numbness in the heel. A similar problem, **stress fracture,** develops in the bones of the foot when extreme stress (running, walking) is continually placed on the ball of the foot.

CAUSES

An **AC separation** results from sudden impact on the side of the shoulder or on an outstretched arm. Wear on the rotator cuff, causing **rotator cuff tendonitis,** may occur if you continually en-gage in sports that require overhead motion like that in a tennis serve. Medial **epicondylitis** is caused by traumatic, repetitive arm motion, as when bowling in cricket. Sudden, violent twisting

---

COMMON SPORTS INJURIES

The highlighted areas below show some of the sites of common injuries sustained from sports or other physi-cal activity. The best way to prevent an athletic injury is to be in good physical condition and to stretch for several minutes before and after exercising. Never at-tempt to 'play through' pain—doing so may cause more extensive injury and lengthen the time needed for complete healing.

SHOULDER JOINT SEPARATION

COLLAR-BONE FRACTURE

SHOULDER DISLOCATION

ROTATOR CUFF TENDONITIS (Back of shoulder)

LUMBAR STRAIN (Lower back)

TENNIS ELBOW (Back of elbow)

QUADRICEPS CONTUSION

JAMMED FINGER

KNEE INJURY

HAMSTRING STRAIN (Back of leg)

SHIN SPLINTS

PATELLAR TENDONITIS

ACHILLES TENDONITIS (Back of ankle)

MUSCLE CRAMPS

STRESS FRACTURE

SPRAINED ANKLE

PLANTAR FASCIITIS (Sole of foot)

of the elbow or continual pulling and strain on the forearm muscles can cause the condition.

Stiffness or **cramp** in the arm or leg is usually caused by a sudden, acute strain in the leg, but mineral deficiency, hormone imbalance, calcium deposits in the muscles, or dehydration can also be causes. Muscle imbalance, a poorly aligned leg, or running on a hard road with improper footwear may cause a **stress fracture.** Tight hamstrings may contribute to lower-back problems, and tight Achilles tendons may precede cases of tendonitis of the foot and ankle.

DIAGNOSTIC AND TEST PROCEDURES

Basic assessment of an injury begins with your medical history and a physical exam. X-rays may be ordered to examine your bones for possible **fractures, dislocations,** and other injuries. A bone scan is a highly sensitive test that may detect **stress fractures** that might not show up in x-rays.

Arthroscopy, ultrasound, and magnetic resonance imaging (MRI) are generally used on joints. Arthroscopy employs a tiny camera inside a very small tube, called an arthroscope, to examine the interior of your joints; it is useful in both diagnosing and repairing some joint injuries (for example, cartilage fragments can be removed through the tube). Ultrasound scanning uses sound waves to generate an image that your doctor can view on a screen. An MRI produces excellent images of soft tissue, enabling diagnosis of damage to muscles, ligaments, and tendons.

TREATMENT

Treatment for sports injuries aims to relieve pain, repair or realign bones, and restore your body to its full athletic ability.

CONVENTIONAL MEDICINE

Most minor soft-tissue injuries are best treated with RICE: rest, ice, compression, and elevation.

Injuries such as tendonitis and **plantar fasciitis** usually require rest and a rehabilitation programme to maintain flexibility and strength. As-

GROWING PAINS

Osgood-Schlatter disease is a condition associated with sudden growth spurts in adolescence (usually in boys ages 10 to 14). It is characterized by pain and swelling below the kneecap, where the patellar tendon attaches to the shinbone. The quadriceps muscle, located at the front of the thigh, continually pulls on the affected tendon, causing the disorder. The condition persists for six months to a year and usually clears up completely without treatment, but as long as your child suffers from symptoms, running, jumping, and squatting should be kept to a minimum, if not eliminated.

pirin or ibuprofen may help reduce the pain and inflammation that accompany these conditions.

Depending on the severity of the pain, your physician may treat your **epicondylitis** with an injection of a corticosteroid, with nonsteroidal anti-inflammatory drugs (NSAIDs) such as ibuprofen, or with aspirin. An elbow cuff and physical therapy may also be indicated.

For acute pain as a result of an **AC separation,** codeine may be prescribed for the first couple of days. Thereafter, aspirin and a nonsteroidal anti-inflammatory drug may be taken for chronic pain. Your physician may immobilize the injured area with a sling.

If possible, the displaced bones of a dislocation are manipulated back into place. If this is not feasible, you may need surgery, after which the joint is immobilized until it is stable.

If necessary, a fracture is treated by reduction, a procedure in which the broken bone ends are manipulated so that they abut each other in their original position. The procedure may be done surgically or without cutting the skin. More serious fractures are repositioned and held in place with metal pins or by screws, plates, and rods placed permanently in or on the bone.

A **stress fracture** is customarily treated by placing the foot in a plaster cast or a rigid boot; you must rest it for three to six weeks.

COMPLEMENTARY CHOICES

ACUPUNCTURE
Administered by a professional, acupuncture may be helpful in treating athletic injuries and soothing the body after strenuous training. It has been shown to reduce pain and swelling and should be applied as soon as possible after injury occurs.

BODY WORK
Massage relieves aches and pains, is especially helpful for tendonitis and **epicondylitis,** and can lessen the onset of muscle soreness. Administered by a professional, the **Alexander technique, Rolfing,** and the **Feldenkrais method** may be useful.

Knead the stiff area of cramping, rubbing in the direction of the muscle fibres.

HOMEOPATHY
Arnica (12c) may be taken every 10 minutes for 1 to 2 hours, until the shock of fracture passes, and then every 8 hours for the next two to three days. Taken every 8 to 12 hours for up to three days, Ruta (12c) may aid healing after a dislocation. The symptoms of a sprained ankle may be eased with Rhus toxicodendron (12c), taken four times a day for as long as a week.

HYDROTHERAPY
Water is the perfect place for athletes recovering from injuries to work out. Aquatic movement provides muscle resistance without straining joints.

LIFESTYLE
Heat before exercise can loosen joints and soft tissue. Various types of braces and supports worn during exercise can protect joints and soft tissue and stabilize an uncomfortable joint or tendon. Consult your doctor or a physical therapist. To avoid ankle injuries, always wear appropriate shoes with ample protection and support.

NUTRITION AND DIET
Many experts advise athletes to maintain a high-carbohydrate, low-fat diet to increase energy levels and promote muscle strength.

Taken orally or topically, vitamin E may guard against muscle damage during exercise. Magnesium helps maintain muscle flexibility, which lessens susceptibility to injury.

For bone fractures, vitamin B complex and zinc may help.

HOME REMEDIES
◆ Replacing fluids lost through perspiration with a carbohydrate-electrolyte sports drink helps prevent cramping.
◆ Ice packs reduce swelling; a bag of frozen vegetables can be a makeshift ice pack. Do not use chemical cold packs; they are much colder than water packs. Place a damp towel around your pack so that it is not directly on your skin.
◆ A warm compress may relieve muscle pain, especially before massage and stretching.
◆ To relieve cramping, elevate the affected area to direct blood flow toward the heart.
◆ If muscles are sore the day after a tough workout, soak in a hot tub and rest the affected area.

PREVENTION

Before you begin a sport or exercise routine, have a physical exam, especially if you are over 40.

Sports injuries usually result when the muscles are poorly conditioned. You should have a 10-minute warmup session—running in place or doing jumping jacks—before an athletic activity to increase your body temperature and diminish chances of muscle injury. Stretching after your workout will help to prevent any soreness the next day.

Engage in your chosen sport or exercise at least three times a week in order to maintain proper conditioning. ■

BACKACHE

SYMPTOMS	AILMENT/PROBLEM
◆ soreness after overexertion or injury; soreness that develops during the night; soreness that radiates to buttocks or thighs.	◆ Back muscle strain
◆ pain, stiffness, and tenderness in the back, buttocks, or thighs; difficulty moving or bending the back.	◆ Osteoarthritis of the spine, also called spondylosis
◆ sudden onset of pain; pain may shoot down one leg after lifting heavy objects, strenuous exercise, twisting, sneezing, or coughing; bending forward at the waist increases pain; lying down eases pain.	◆ Herniated disc (also called prolapsed disc); ruptured disc; or slipped disc
◆ chronic low-back pain that comes and goes for months or years.	◆ Misalignment of the spine
◆ sharp pain in a specific place along the spine.	◆ Osteoporosis
◆ pain in the lower back in a woman who is more than four months pregnant.	◆ Pregnancy problem
◆ pain in the lower back; fever of 38°C or above; painful urination; nausea or vomiting.	◆ Kidney infection
◆ chronic pain and stiffness that seem worse in the morning; person with the pain is between the ages of 20 and 40.	◆ Ankylosing spondylitis
◆ pain in back, buttocks, thighs, and/or calves when walking or climbing stairs; pain is relieved by standing still or sitting.	◆ Spinal stenosis
◆ back pain, especially at night, that is unrelieved by lying down.	◆ Possibly, a tumour

WHAT TO DO	OTHER INFO
◆ Rest for a few days; use pain relievers if necessary.	◆ Physical therapy may include the application of heat and cold, gentle massage, and exercises to prevent future problems.
◆ See Arthritis. Take an anti-inflammatory drug for pain relief. Rest, heat, exercise, and physical therapy may be helpful.	◆ This condition may be caused by strain, injury, or ageing.
◆ Treatment may include pain relievers, bed rest, physical therapy, and wearing a supportive collar.	◆ Disc problems may lead to other problems, such as sciatica or bowel or bladder incontinence. Osteopathy and acupuncture may help. If part of the disc is pressing on a nerve, surgery may, as a last resort, be needed.
◆ Call your doctor.	◆ The underlying cause may be poor muscle tone in the abdomen or back, obesity, or osteoarthritis.
◆ Hormone replacement therapy may be recommended for postmenopausal women, to prevent further bone loss.	◆ This condition is most common in women over 60 and people confined to bed or a wheelchair. Patients are encouraged not to smoke or drink alcohol, to eat less animal protein and fat, to obtain sufficient calcium, and to do weight-bearing exercise.
◆ Learning how to lift properly, wearing supportive shoes, improving posture, and sleeping on a firm mattress may help.	◆ Acupressure, massage, or osteopathy may be helpful.
◆ **Call your doctor now.** A kidney infection requires immediate treatment with antibiotics.	◆ Be sure to take the antibiotics for the full length of the prescription.
◆ Usual treatment is anti-inflammatory drugs, physical therapy, massage, and prescribed exercises.	◆ Treatment is essential to prevent progression to fusion of the joints and a rigid spine.
◆ Call your doctor. Losing weight and doing abdominal exercises may help. Surgery is required in some cases.	◆ The pain is caused by a narrowing of the spinal canal at a point where a nerve passes. Modifying the posture may help.
◆ **Call your doctor without delay.** A medical evaluation is necessary for diagnosis and treatment.	◆ A tumour may be benign or malignant. By the time it causes pain, it is probably sizable. Cancer of the back is more likely in someone who already has cancer elsewhere.

- a burning sensation when urinating; this is the most common sign of a bladder infection, but any pain or difficulty in urination may also indicate the condition.
- frequent urge to urinate.
- urine with a strong, foul odour.
- in the elderly: lethargy, incontinence, mental confusion.

In severe cases, these symptoms may be accompanied by fever and chills, abdominal pain, or blood in the urine.

CALL YOUR DOCTOR IF:

- the burning sensation persists for more than 24 hours after you begin trying self-help treatments. Untreated, bladder infections can lead to more serious conditions.
- painful urination is accompanied by vomiting, fever, chills, bloody urine, or abdominal or back pain; it may indicate potentially life-threatening kidney disease, a bladder or kidney tumour, or prostate infection. **Seek medical help immediately.**
- the burning is accompanied by a discharge from the vagina or penis, a sign of sexually transmitted disease, pelvic inflammatory disease (PID), or other serious infection. See your doctor without delay.
- you experience any persistent pain or difficulty with urination; this may also be a sign of sexually transmitted disease, a vaginal infection, a kidney stone, enlargement of the prostate, or a bladder or prostate tumour. See your doctor without delay.

Bladder infections—generally termed cystitis, which means inflammation of the bladder—are common in women and very rare in men. In fact, about half of all women get at least one bladder infection at some time in their lives. Although doctors are not sure exactly why women have many more bladder infections than men, they suspect it may be because women have a shorter urethra, the tube that carries urine out of the bladder. This relatively short passageway—only about 4 centimetres long—makes it easier for bacteria to migrate into the bladder. Also, the opening to a woman's urethra lies close to both the vagina and the anus, giving bacteria from those areas access to the urinary tract.

Bladder infections are not serious if treated promptly. But recurrences are common in susceptible people and can lead to kidney infections, which are more serious and may result in permanent kidney damage. So it's very important to treat the underlying causes of a bladder infection and to take preventive steps to avoid recurrences.

In elderly people, bladder infections are often difficult to diagnose because the symptoms are less specific and are frequently blamed on ageing. Older people who suddenly become incontinent or who begin acting lethargic or confused should be checked by a doctor for a bladder infection.

CAUSES

Most bladder infections are caused by various strains of *Escherichia coli (E. coli),* the bacteria commonly found in the intestines. Women sometimes get bladder infections as a direct result of intercourse, which can push bacteria up into the bladder through the urethra. Some women contract the infection—dubbed 'honeymoon cystitis'—almost every time they have sex. Women who use a diaphragm as their primary method of birth control are also particularly susceptible to bladder infections, perhaps because the device presses on the bladder and keeps it from emptying completely. Bacteria then rapidly reproduce in the stagnant urine left in the bladder. Pregnant women, whose bladders become compressed as the fetus grows, are prone to infections for the same reason. Some people develop symptoms of a bladder infection when no infection actually exists. These disorders are usually benign but are difficult to treat.

While they can be quite uncomfortable and potentially serious if complications set in, the bladder infections that most women get clear up quickly and are relatively harmless. In men, however, a bladder infection is almost always a symptom of an underlying disorder and is generally regarded as cause for more concern. Often the infection has migrated from the prostate or some other part of the body, signalling problems in those locations. Or it may indicate the presence of a tumour or other obstruction that is interfering with the urinary tract. Some studies have shown that uncircumcised boys are at somewhat greater risk of contracting a bladder infection during their first year of life because bacteria may collect under the foreskin.

In recent years, an increasing number of bladder infections in both men and women have been linked to two sexually transmitted bacteria, chlamydia and mycoplasma. And both home and hospital use of catheters—tubes inserted into the bladder to empty it—can also lead to infection.

DIAGNOSTIC AND TEST PROCEDURES

Bladder infections usually can be diagnosed readily with a urine test. If you are experiencing persistent or frequent infections, or if an anatomical defect is suspected as the cause of the problem, your physician may also want you to undergo cystoscopy, a diagnostic procedure in which a lighted tube inserted through the urethra is used to examine the inside of the bladder. And to make sure your kidneys have not been affected, your physician may order an intravenous pyelogram (IVP), a special x-ray technique for viewing kidneys, or an ultrasound scan to produce an image of the entire urinary tract system.

TREATMENT

Mild bladder infections often clear up quickly in response to simple home remedies. But if you ex-
perience no relief within 24 hours, you should consult a physician for more aggressive treatment. Delay in clearing your body of the infection can lead to more serious problems.

CONVENTIONAL MEDICINE

Bladder infections are treated with a wide variety of antibiotics to clear up the infection; with strong prescription painkillers to relieve the pain and burning; and by increased intake of fluids to flush out the urinary tract. The antibiotic your physician prescribes and the number of days you will need to take it will depend on the type of bacteria that are causing the infection. Although some studies indicate that uncomplicated infections require only one to three days of treatment, your physician may prefer to treat you for a longer period of time in order to ensure that all of the bacteria are eradicated. Elderly people and those with a chronic underlying health condition, such as diabetes or HIV infection, are often prescribed a longer course of antibiotics— sometimes up to 14 days.

After the treatment has run its course, you may be asked to come in for a follow-up urine test to make sure your bladder is free of all.signs of infection. People with frequently recurring bladder infections are often prescribed low daily doses of antibiotics for an additional six months or longer. Patients whose infections are related to sexual activity may be given a small dose of antibiotics to take each time they have intercourse. Some doctors prescribe the hormone oestrogen, either as a topical cream or in pill form, to prevent recurrences in postmenopausal women. For cases where the infection is the result of a blockage or obstruction, such as a kidney stone or an enlarged prostate, surgery may be required.

COMPLEMENTARY CHOICES

If begun promptly at the first hint of burning during urination, alternative means of treatment can be successful in getting rid of a bladder infection. But if these methods do not bring relief within 24 hours, you should call your doctor for antibiotic treatment. Consult with your doctor if you wish to continue with alternative methods while on the antibiotics to speed up the recovery process.

ACUPUNCTURE

Acupuncture treatment may help prevent recurrences of bladder infections. Consult a professional acupuncturist.

CHIROPRACTIC/OSTEOPATHY

Adjusting the bones and joints around the pelvis can act to strengthen the bladder muscles, helping to ward off recurrences of the infection. An **osteopath** can also provide this treatment.

HERBAL THERAPIES

Some herbs have been found useful in both clearing up bladder infections and easing the burning that accompanies them. Perhaps the best known is cranberry, which, recent scientific studies show, has a remarkable ability to combat bladder and other urinary tract infections *(box, opposite).*

Another herb useful in treating bladder infections is nettle *(Urtica dioica),* which has been shown to have anti-inflammatory properties. Mix 1 tsp dried, crushed nettle leaves or root in 1 cup boiling water. Allow the infusion to cool, then drink 1 tbsp every hour or two—up to 1 cup a day.

The evergreen shrub uva ursi *(Arctostaphylos uva-ursi),* or bearberry, which acts as a diuretic and an anti-inflammatory medication, has a long history as a folk remedy for bladder infections. Soak fresh leaves in brandy or other liquor for a few hours, then add to boiling water—about 1 tsp leaves per cup of water. If you have dried leaves, you can boil them directly in the water without a preliminary alcohol soak.

Women who are prone to bladder infections after sexual activity can help prevent recurrences by washing their perineal area with a medicinal solution of the herb goldenseal *(Hydrastis canadensis)* before and after intercourse. Mix 2 tsp of the herb per cup of water, bring to a boil, and simmer for 15 minutes. Cool to room temperature before using.

HOMEOPATHY

Depending on the symptoms, homeopaths recommend a number of different remedies to help relieve the pain of a bladder infection. Here are three of the most commonly prescribed:
- If the urge to urinate is very strong and the burning is intense, Cantharis.
- If you experience painful cramping with urination or your urine is very dark or bloody, Mercurius corrosivus.
- For women whose infections are brought on by sexual contact, Staphysagria.

Take these remedies hourly until symptoms disappear. If you experience no relief after 24 hours, seek professional help.

HYDROTHERAPY AND AROMATHERAPY

Hot sitz baths can help relieve the symptoms of a bladder infection. Adding certain pungent herbal oils to the bathwater creates a soothing, fragrant steam that aromatherapists believe makes the treatment particularly effective. Try putting in a few drops of the essential oils of juniper berry, eucalyptus, sandalwood, pine, parsley, cedarwood, chamomile, or cajuput.

You can also try a massage oil made with 30 ml vegetable oil and 5 drops each of any com-

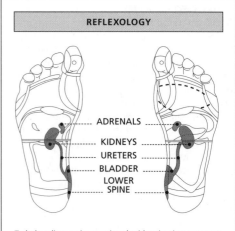

REFLEXOLOGY

ADRENALS
KIDNEYS
URETERS
BLADDER
LOWER SPINE

To help relieve pain associated with urination, use your left thumb to work the areas on your right foot that correspond to the adrenals, kidneys, ureters, bladder, and lower spine. Repeat on the left foot.

ily spiced dishes. Wait 10 days after the burning is gone before reintroducing these foods and drinks—one at a time—into your diet.

Supplements of vitamin C (500 mg every two hours) and vitamin A (25,000 IU each day) may also aid recovery. But check with your doctor before taking the supplements. Vitamin C increases the acidity of urine, which hampers the growth of bacteria but can also interfere with the action of some antibiotics, making them less effective.

HOME REMEDIES
◆ Take aspirin or ibuprofen to reduce inflammation and burning.
◆ Drink cranberry juice daily.

PREVENTION

◆ Practise good bathroom hygiene. Clean the anal area thoroughly after a bowel movement. Women should wipe from front to back to avoid spreading faecal bacteria to the urethra.
◆ Urinate as soon as possible when you feel the urge, and make sure you empty your bladder completely each time.
◆ Wear cotton underwear and loose, nonbinding clothing that does not trap heat and moisture in the crotch.
◆ Drink plenty of liquids.

Women:
◆ Empty your bladder as soon as possible after intercourse to wash out any bacteria that may have been pushed into the urethra.
◆ Avoid using perfumed soaps, bubble baths, scented douches, and vaginal deodorants. These contain substances that can irritate the urethra and make it more vulnerable to infection.
◆ If you use a diaphragm for birth control, make sure it fits properly, and don't leave it in for longer than you have been instructed. ■

bination of the herbs mentioned. Massage daily, rubbing the oil over your lower back, abdomen, stomach, and hips.

NUTRITION AND DIET
Both conventional and alternative practitioners agree that drinking plenty of fluids to keep you urinating frequently and to flush out your urinary tract thoroughly is one of the most effective means of combating a bladder infection—whatever its cause. However, you should avoid beverages that might irritate the urinary tract and aggravate the burning. Culprits include alcohol, coffee, black tea, chocolate milk, carbonated beverages, and citrus juices. Until clear of the infection, you should also avoid potentially irritating foods such as citrus fruits, tomatoes, vinegar, sugar, chocolate, artificial sweeteners, and heav-

BOWEL MOVEMENT ABNORMALITIES

Read down this column to find your symptoms. Then read across.

SYMPTOMS	AILMENT/PROBLEM
◆ passing hard and/or infrequent stools or straining to have a bowel movement.	◆ Constipation
◆ watery and/or frequent bowel movements.	◆ Diarrhoea
◆ worms in the stool, perhaps appearing as light-coloured threads; possible itching in the anal area.	◆ Pinworm, roundworm, or tapeworm infection
◆ alternating hard/infrequent and watery/frequent stools.	◆ Irritable bowel syndrome; colon tumour; diabetes; alternating use of laxatives and antidiarrhoeal drugs
◆ extremely foul-smelling, large stools; weight loss despite good appetite; abdominal pain.	◆ Pancreatic problems, possibly associated with coeliac disease
◆ any visible blood in the stools.	◆ Many possibilities, including haemorrhoids, anal fissure, and colorectal cancer
◆ persistent thin, ribbonlike stools; possible anal bleeding.	◆ Possibly, colorectal cancer
◆ maroon-colored or black, tarry, metallic-smelling stools; possible abdominal pain.	◆ Bleeding from the upper or middle gastro-intestinal tract, caused by any of a number of ailments or use of certain medications
◆ stools that are either too hard or too watery; abdominal pain; flatulence; nausea; vomiting; fever.	◆ Appendicitis
◆ black or dark-red stools; vomiting with blood; easy bruising; spiderlike blood vessels on the skin; fatigue; yellowish skin and eyes; weight loss or gain; distended abdomen.	◆ Cirrhosis
◆ pale or chalky stools; dark-orange to tea-coloured urine; yellowish skin and eyes; dull abdominal pain, fever, shaking, chills.	◆ Bile duct blocked by a gallstone; gall-bladder disorder; liver disorder

|

WHAT TO DO	OTHER INFO
◆ Change to a high-fibre diet and drink at least eight glasses of water each day.	◆ Over 30 possible causes, including: irritable bowel, anal fissure, depression, and inactivity.
◆ Drink fluids copiously to replace those being lost. If diarrhoea persists beyond 48 hours, call your doctor.	◆ More than a dozen causes, including flu and food poisoning.
◆ See your doctor; prescription medication can cure the infection.	◆ Wormwood (Artemisia absinthium) taken three times daily in a pill or a tea (pour 1 cup boiling water over $1/2$ tsp wormwood; steep for 10 minutes) is reported to cure many worm infestations.
◆ If you frequently use laxatives and anti-diarrhoeal drugs, gradually reduce your use until you can stop; otherwise, call your doctor without delay for proper diagnosis.	◆ Laxatives can mimic the abdominal pain of irritable bowel syndrome or a colon tumour.
◆ See your doctor soon. You may need to eliminate all gluten-containing foods from your diet.	◆ If coeliac disease prevents absorption of iron, vitamin B_{12}, or folic acid, take supplements.
◆ Call your doctor today—immediately if patient is a child or if bleeding is profuse.	◆ Never ignore anal bleeding; it can indicate colorectal cancer.
◆ Call your doctor today; an early and accurate diagnosis is essential.	◆ Treated early, colorectal cancer is curable; untreated, it can be fatal.
◆ Call your doctor today for a proper diagnosis; report any prescription or over-the-counter medications you are taking.	◆ A home test kit can determine if blood is in stools; maroon colour may be from eating red foods such as beetroots.
◆ **Call your doctor or seek emergency care now — call 999.**	
◆ **Call your doctor or seek emergency medical help now — call 999;** cirrhosis may be life-threatening.	◆ Avoid alcohol, high-fat foods, and all drugs (except those your doctor prescribes) to enhance liver function.
◆ Adopt a low-fat diet. If abdominal pain is severe or any fever is present, see your doctor immediately.	◆ Vitamin K supplements may help alleviate symptoms.

Acute Bronchitis:
- hacking cough.
- yellow, white, or green phlegm, usually appearing 24 to 48 hours after a cough.
- fever, chills.
- soreness and tightness in chest.
- some pain below breastbone during deep breathing.

Chronic Bronchitis:
- persistent cough producing yellow, white, or green phlegm (for at least three months of the year, and for more than two consecutive years).
- wheezing, some breathlessness.

CALL YOUR DOCTOR IF:

- ◆ your cough is so persistent or severe that it interferes with sleep or daily activities; you could be damaging sensitive air sacs in your lungs.
- ◆ your symptoms last more than a week, and your mucus becomes darker, thicker, or increases in volume; most likely, you have an infection requiring antibiotics.
- ◆ you display symptoms of acute bronchitis and have chronic lung or heart problems or are infected with the virus that causes AIDS; respiratory infections can leave you vulnerable to more serious lung diseases, such as pneumonia.
- ◆ you have great difficulty breathing. This symptom, sometimes mistakenly associated with bronchitis, could signal asthma, emphysema, tuberculosis, heart disease, a serious allergic reaction, or cancer.

Bronchitis is an upper respiratory disease in which the mucous membrane in the lungs' upper bronchial passages becomes inflamed. As the irritated membrane swells and grows thicker, it narrows or shuts off the tiny airways in the lungs, resulting in coughing spells accompanied by thick phlegm and breathlessness. The disease comes in two forms: acute and chronic.

Acute bronchitis is responsible for the hacking cough and phlegm production that sometimes accompany an upper respiratory infection; in most cases the infection is viral in origin, but sometimes it is caused by bacteria. If you are otherwise in good health, the mucous membrane will return to normal after you've recovered from the initial lung infection, which usually lasts for several days.

Chronic bronchitis, like the lung disease emphysema, is a serious long-term disorder that requires regular medical treatment. People who have chronic bronchitis tend to be obese and lead sedentary lives, and most are heavy smokers; they typically have emphysema as well, which accounts for some of the overlapping symptoms.

If you are a smoker and come down with acute bronchitis, it will be much harder for you to recover. Even one puff on a cigarette is enough to cause temporary paralysis of the tiny hairlike cells in your lungs that are responsible for brushing out debris, irritants, and excess mucus. If you continue smoking, you may do sufficient damage to these cells, known as cilia, to prevent them from functioning properly, thus increasing your chances of developing chronic bronchitis. In some heavy smokers, the membrane stays inflamed and the cilia eventually stop functioning altogether. Clogged with mucus, the lungs are then vulnerable to viral and bacterial infections, which over time distort and permanently damage the lungs' airways.

Acute bronchitis is very common among both children and adults. Although the disorder often can be treated effectively without professional medical assistance, you will need to see a doctor for a prescription of antibiotics if the underlying lung infection is bacterial. If you suffer from **chronic bronchitis,** you are at risk of developing cardiovascular problems as well as more serious lung diseases and infections, so you should be monitored by a doctor.

CAUSES

Acute bronchitis is generally caused by lung infections; approximately 90 per cent of these infections are viral in origin, 10 per cent bacterial. **Chronic bronchitis** may be caused by one or several factors. Repeated attacks of acute bronchitis, which weaken and irritate bronchial airways over time, can result in chronic bronchitis. Industrial pollution is another culprit. Chronic bronchitis is found in higher than normal rates among coal miners, grain handlers, metalworkers, and other people who are continually exposed to dust. But the chief cause is heavy, long-term cigarette smoking, which irritates the bronchial tubes and causes them to produce excess mucus. The symptoms of chronic bronchitis are also worsened by high concentrations of sulphur dioxide and other pollutants in the atmosphere.

DIAGNOSTIC AND TEST PROCEDURES

Tests are usually unnecessary in the case of **acute bronchitis,** as the disease is easy to detect on examination. Your doctor will simply use a stethoscope to listen for the rattling sound in your lungs' upper airways that typically accompanies the problem. If your symptoms persist for a week or more, your doctor may also take a culture of the phlegm you produce when you cough, to determine if you have a bacterial or viral infection. In cases of **chronic bronchitis,** the doctor will almost certainly augment these procedures with an x-ray of your chest to check the extent of the lung damage, as well as with pulmonary function tests to measure your lung capacity.

TREATMENT

Conventional treatment for both acute and chronic bronchitis may consist of antibiotics and a prescription cough syrup. In severe cases of chronic bronchitis, supplemental oxygen may be

THE BRONCHIAL TUBES

NORMAL BRONCHIAL TUBE
MUCOUS MEMBRANE
CLOGGED BRONCHIAL TUBE
EXCESS MUCUS

Air flows down the windpipe and into the lungs through branching conduits called the bronchial tubes, or bronchioles, which normally are lined with only a thin mucous membrane. In bronchitis, however, this membrane becomes inflamed, resulting in stepped-up mucus production. Over time, excess mucus can clog the bronchioles, cutting off air flow to the lungs. Coughing is the body's way of ridding the lungs of this mucus buildup.

necessary. Complementary choices, by and large, help relieve the accompanying discomfort but do not treat infections.

CONVENTIONAL MEDICINE

If your **acute bronchitis** is caused by a bacterial infection, your doctor probably will prescribe antibiotics, which should help clear up the symptoms in several days. Even if the cause is viral, your doctor may prescribe antibiotics as a preventive measure, because your lungs are susceptible to bacterial infections in their weakened state. The productive (phlegm-producing) coughing that comes with acute bronchitis is to be expected and, in most cases, encouraged; coughing is your body's way of getting rid of excess mucus. However, if your cough is truly disruptive—that is, it keeps you from sleeping or is so violent it becomes painful—or nonproductive (dry and raspy sounding), your doctor may prescribe a cough suppressant. In most cases, you should simply do all the things you normally would do for a cold: Take aspirin for fever and drink lots of liquids.

If you have **chronic bronchitis,** your lungs are

vulnerable to infections. Unless your doctor counsels against it, get a yearly flu injection as well as a vaccination against pneumonia. The pneumonia vaccine is typically a one-shot procedure: One vaccination should protect you for life against all the common strains of the disease. Only in very rare cases is a second injection required.

Do not take an over-the-counter cough suppressant to treat chronic bronchitis unless your doctor directs you to do so. As with acute bronchitis, the productive coughing associated with chronic bronchitis is helpful in ridding the lungs of excess mucus. In fact, your doctor may even prescribe an expectorant if your cough is relatively dry. However, if you notice any changes in the colour, volume, or thickness of the phlegm, you may be coming down with an infection. In that case, your doctor may prescribe a week-long or 10-day course of broad-spectrum antibiotics, which fight a range of bacteria.

If you are overweight, your doctor may insist that you diet to avoid putting excessive strain on your heart. Many doctors also prescribe bronchodilators, drugs that help dilate the lungs' constricted airways. For people with chronic bronchitis, inhaled bronchodilators, available in aerosol or metered-dose inhalers, are generally preferred over oral medications. In most cases, one or two puffs will relieve the breathlessness that accompanies chronic bronchitis. Special circumstances may require a greater dosage, but you should never increase your intake unless instructed to do so by your doctor. Bronchodilators are potent drugs; overuse can cause dangerous side effects, such as high blood pressure.

If your body's ability to transfer oxygen from your lungs into the bloodstream is significantly handicapped, your doctor may prescribe **oxygen therapy,** either on a continuous or on an as-needed basis. Oxygen-delivering devices are widely available. If you use an oxygen tank at home, be sure to take special care not to expose the apparatus to flammable materials (alcohol and aerosol sprays, for example) or to sources of direct heat, such as hair dryers or radiators.

If you smoke, your doctor will urge you to quit. Studies show that people who kick the habit even in the advanced stages of chronic bronchitis not only can reduce the severity of their symptoms but can also increase their life expectancy.

ALTERNATIVE CHOICES

A number of alternative therapies can be used to complement—but never to replace—a conventional doctor's care. These remedies may help ease some of the symptoms of acute and chronic bronchitis, but they do not treat infections.

ACUPUNCTURE

Studies suggest that acupuncture may relieve the symptoms associated with bronchitis. The technique should be performed only by a licensed acupuncturist.

AROMATHERAPY

Essential oils such as eucalyptus *(Eucalyptus globulus),* hyssop *(Hyssopus officinalis),* aniseed *(Pimpinella anisum),* lavender *(Lavandula officinalis),* pine *(Pinus sylvestris),* and rosemary *(Rosmarinus officinalis)* may help ease breathing and relieve nasal congestion. Inhaling deeply through your nose, breathe the aroma from a few drops of one or more of these oils dabbed on a handkerchief, or sniff directly from the bottle. Try mixing a few drops of essential oil in a sink full of hot water; cover your head with a towel and breathe in the fragrant steam.

CHINESE HERBS

The Chinese herb ephedra *(Ephedra sinica)* is a potent bronchodilator. CAUTION: Large quantities of this herb have the same effect as large quantities of the hormone adrenaline; do not use ephedra if you have high blood pressure or heart disease. Prepare an infusion by combining 5 grams ephedra, 4 grams cinnamon sticks *(Cinnamomum cassia),* 1.5 grams licorice *(Glycyrrhiza glabra),* and 5 grams apricot seed *(Prunus armeniaca).* Steep the mixture in cold water, then bring it to a boil. Drink it hot.

HERBAL THERAPIES

A wide variety of herbs act as soothing expectorants, making them appropriate in the treatment of bronchitis. A sampling of therapies follows; for more, seek the advice of a professional herbalist or homeopath.

In the case of **acute** or **chronic bronchitis,** the herb coltsfoot *(Tussilago farfara)* may relax constricted or spasming bronchial tubes and gently help to loosen phlegm. To prepare an infusion, add a cup of boiling water to 1 or 2 tsp of coltsfoot; let the infusion steep for 10 minutes. Drink it as hot as possible, three times daily. Mullein *(Verbascum thapsus),* believed to have an anti-inflammatory effect on mucous membranes, can also be prepared as an infusion by following the directions above.

To treat **acute bronchitis,** use the same directions to prepare an infusion from the herb hyssop *(Hyssopus officinalis),* which may encourage sweating (thus lowering fever) and lessen inflammation. Herbal expectorants appropriate for **chronic bronchitis** include aniseed/anise *(Pimpinella anisum),* elecampane *(Inula helenium),* and garlic *(Allium sativum).*

HOMEOPATHY

For **acute** and **chronic bronchitis,** take the following three times a day, for up to four days: To treat fever, cough, and tightness in the chest, use Aconite (6c). For loose white phlegm, cough, and irritability, use Kali bichromicum (6c). For loss of voice, cough, thirst, and sore throat, use Phosphorus (6c).

NUTRITION AND DIET

To strengthen the immune system and protect against infection, nutritionists often recommend vitamins A, B complex, C, and E, along with the minerals selenium and zinc. Some experts suggest that you also avoid mucus-producing foods, found mainly in the dairy group (although goat's milk generally causes less mucus production than cow's milk), as well as in refined starches (white-flour–based products) and processed foods.

HOME REMEDIES
For acute bronchitis:
Throughout the duration of your infection, stay at home and keep warm. You don't necessarily need to stay in bed, but don't overextend yourself. Consider using a vaporizer, or try inhaling steam over a sink or bowl full of hot water with a cloth over your head and the bowl.

For chronic bronchitis:
Avoid exposure to paint or exhaust fumes, dust, and people with colds. Consider using a vaporizer or inhaling steam over a sink or bowl full of hot water, with a cloth over your head and the bowl. Dress warmly in cold, dry weather. ■

Steaming TOWARD RECOVERY

Humidity is helpful in treating both acute and chronic bronchitis, as moisture in the air can loosen phlegm inside the lungs and make it easier for you to expectorate. To be effective, however, humidifying devices must be used properly.

The warm steam distributed by vaporizers works well when used in a relatively small space, such as a bathroom; in an average-size room, most vaporizers aren't powerful enough to generate the density of steam necessary to be truly helpful. Be sure to clean the vaporizer regularly for the duration of your infection, to prevent the distribution of germs.

Some devices can actually be hazardous to your health. Cold humidifiers, used frequently in homes with dry air, must be cleaned daily with bleach; otherwise, they can spread germs and encourage mould or mildew growth, increasing your chances of developing lung infections.

SYMPTOMS

- a very itchy rash that spreads from the torso to the neck, face, and limbs. The rash, lasting 7 to 10 days, progresses from red spots to fluid-filled blisters (vesicles) that drain and scab over. Vesicles may also appear in the mouth, around the eyes, or on the genitals, and can be very painful.

CALL YOUR DOCTOR IF:

- you think your child has chickenpox; a doctor can confirm your diagnosis.
- chickenpox is accompanied by severe skin pain, and the rash produces a greenish discharge and looks inflamed—signs of a secondary bacterial skin infection.
- chickenpox-is accompanied by a stiff neck, persistent sleepiness, or lethargy—symptoms of acute encephalitis, a serious illness. **Get medical help immediately.**
- your child is recovering from chickenpox and begins running a fever, vomiting, has convulsions, or is somnolent; these are signs of Reye's syndrome, a dangerous, potentially fatal disease that sometimes follows viral infections, particularly if aspirin has been used in treatment. **Get medical help immediately.**
- an adult family member gets chickenpox; in adults, the illness can lead to complications such as pneumonia. See your doctor without delay.
- you are pregnant, have never had chickenpox, and are exposed to the disease; your unborn child may be at risk for birth defects. See your doctor without delay.

Chickenpox, a viral illness characterized by a very itchy red rash, is one of the most common infectious diseases of childhood. It is usually mild in children, but adults run the risk of serious complications, such as bacterial pneumonia.

People who have had chickenpox develop lifetime immunity. But the virus remains dormant in the body, and if you had chickenpox as a child, you may later develop shingles. Because chickenpox can pass from a pregnant woman to her unborn child, possibly causing birth defects, doctors often advise women considering pregnancy to confirm their immunity with a blood test.

CAUSES

Chickenpox is caused by the varicella zoster virus. This virus may lie dormant and manifest itself in adult life as herpes zoster or shingles. It is spread by droplets from a sneeze or cough, or by

IDENTIFYING THE RASH

Small, red bumps appear on the chest and back and soon form a rash of itchy, fluid-filled blisters that burst and form scabs. Within days the rash spreads to the face, arms, and legs (right). Scabs will dry and drop off about a week after they appear, and the rash should be gone in two weeks. Avoid scratching the scabs; they may become infected and leave scars if scratched.

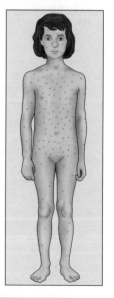

contact with the clothing, bed linens, or oozing vesicles of an infected person. The incubation period is 7 to 21 days; the disease is most contagious a day before the rash appears and up to 7 days after, or until the rash forms scabs.

TREATMENT

Chickenpox is extremely contagious. Keep your child at home until most of the vesicles are dry and the scabs have fallen off.

CONVENTIONAL MEDICINE

Your doctor may prescribe an antihistamine, to relieve pain and swelling. Antibiotics are called for if a secondary bacterial skin infection arises or if an adult with chickenpox contracts bacterial pneumonia. Acyclovir, an antiviral drug, is sometimes prescribed in severe cases, although some doctors question its effectiveness.

COMPLEMENTARY CHOICES

HERBAL THERAPIES

For itching, herbalists recommend the following wash: Add 1 oz each dried rosemary (Rosmarinus officinalis) and calendula (Calendula officinalis) to a good litre of water. Bring to a boil, then simmer for five minutes. Strain, discard the herbs, and allow the wash to cool. Press a washcloth dampened in the solution to the child's skin after a bath. The wash can be reused for three days if refrigerated.

HOMEOPATHY

Consult a homeopath for appropriate remedies and dosages for children. To relieve itching, your practitioner may prescribe Rhus toxicodendron, especially if itching is worse at night. Sulphur may help when the vesicles are burning.

HOME REMEDIES

◆ Trim your child's fingernails or cover her hands with socks or mittens to keep her from scratching, which could lead to infection as well as to possible scarring.
◆ To ease itching, add a handful of oatmeal or baking soda to bathwater; apply cool, wet towels to the skin and allow them to dry.
◆ Dab calamine or witch hazel on the lesions to relieve itching. Do not use lotions containing diphenhydramine, which may sensitize your child to antihistamines.
◆ Leave your baby's nappy off as much as possible to allow the vesicles to dry out and form scabs.
◆ Dissolve ½ tsp salt in a glass of warm water and use as a gargle to ease mouth ulcers.

PREVENTION

Some doctors now recommend that children be immunized, usually after the child is a year old, as a protection to vulnerable people such as pregnant women. Consult your family doctor for advice.

PREGNANCY CONCERNS

If you have not had chickenpox and are exposed to the virus while pregnant, contact your doctor immediately. A varicella zoster immunoglobulin injection, given within 72 hours of exposure, may help lessen the severity of the disease. The virus can still pass to your unborn child through the umbilical cord, but possible complications such as fetal malformation or retarded growth may be less likely to occur. If you give birth while you have chickenpox, the baby should also receive immunoglobulin.

C A U T I O N !

Never give aspirin—even baby aspirin—or other products containing the salt called salicylate to a child who has chickenpox. Aspirin has been linked to Reye's syndrome, a rare but very dangerous illness that causes inflammation of the liver and brain. ∎

SYMPTOMS

- head and chest congestion, perhaps with a runny nose and difficulty breathing.
- sore throat.
- sneezing.
- dry cough that may occur only at night.
- chills.
- burning, watery eyes.
- vague aches all over.
- headache.
- constant fatigue.

CALL YOUR DOCTOR IF:

- your newborn (two months or younger) has cold symptoms. For infants, the common cold can be a serious illness.
- congestion makes it hard to breathe, or your chest makes a whistling sound (a wheeze) when you breathe. You may have asthma.
- your throat hurts and your temperature is over 38°C or higher; or your cold symptoms worsen after the third day. You may have a bacterial infection (such as streptococcus), sinusitis, or bronchitis.
- your temperature is over 39°C or higher. You may have pneumonia. **Seek medical care immediately.**
- your cold symptoms occur suddenly with exposure to certain triggers—such as pollen, cats, or perfume—and/or the symptoms continue for weeks. You probably have an allergy.

The aptly named common cold is the most frequent infection in all age groups. Cold symptoms are triggered when a virus attaches itself to the lining of your nasal passages or throat. Your immune system responds by attacking the germ with white blood cells. If your immune system cannot recognize the virus, the response is 'nonspecific', meaning your body produces as many white blood cells as possible (usually more than are needed) and circulates them to the infected sites. This all-out attack kills many viruses, but it doesn't affect the 200 or so viruses that cause colds. Extra white blood cells clumping together at infection sites is what causes the achiness and inflammation of a cold, complete with vast amounts of mucus in the nose and throat.

Cold symptoms settle in between one and four days after you are infected by a cold virus and typically last for about three days. At that point the worst is over, but you may feel congested for a week or more. During the first three days that you have symptoms, you are contagious (meaning you can pass the cold to others), so take preventive measures. *(See Prevention, page 83.)*

Although everyone catches colds, children have them more often than adults. Cold infections are most common during the autumn and winter. During this time of the year people are more likely to congregate indoors, usually with some form of central heating on. Closer contact with others, which increases your chances of being exposed to contagious viruses, and hot, dry air, which dries the nose and throat tissues, help create a perfect environment for a viral infection.

Except in newborns, colds themselves are not dangerous. They usually go away in a week or so without any special medicine. Unfortunately, colds do wear down your body's resistance, making you more susceptible to bacterial infections.

CAUSES

More than 200 viruses can infect your nose and throat and cause the common cold. Unfortunately, there is no absolute cure for any of them, so determining which one is causing your cold won't help you recover any quicker. You 'catch' a cold virus by breathing minute, airborne droplets from a cold sufferer's cough or sneeze, or, more rarely, by touching a virus-infected surface—such as a doorknob or telephone—and then transferring the germs to your nose or mouth.

DIAGNOSTIC AND TEST PROCEDURES

If your cold is nasty enough to send you to the doctor, she will probably examine your throat and ears and may take a throat culture (brushing your throat with a long cotton-tipped swab) to determine if you have a bacterial infection, which requires treatment with antibiotics.

TREATMENT

Conventional and complementary medicine seek the same ends: to make it as easy as possible for your body to fight the cold virus while alleviating the aches and congestion as much as possible. Adequate rest and sleep is key to cold recovery; you may find you need 12 hours or more of sleep per night while you're fighting the cold. Drinking water is also important. Mucus flows freely in a well-hydrated body, helping you avoid or recover from infection; and healthy, moist tissues are harder for a virus to infect than dry tissues. If you have a fever, your body is using heat to help kill the cold virus. Giving medication to lower a fever can actually undermine your body's defence efforts. A temperature of over 39°C or higher warrants a call to your doctor, however.

Pregnant or nursing mothers should check with their doctor before using any type of cold therapy whatsoever, including over-the-counter drugs and herbal remedies.

CONVENTIONAL MEDICINE

No specific treatment exists for the virus that is causing your cold, but in treating your symptoms you can find relief. Ibuprofen can relieve aches, but paracetamol and aspirin may make congestion worse. Never give aspirin to a child with a fever; give paracetamol instead (see Caution below). If your throat is sore, gargle as often as you like with salt water (½ tsp salt in 1 cup water).

It's tempting to acquiesce to an advertiser's claims and try one of the many over-the-counter cold and flu preparations, but think twice. These multisymptom drugs are likely to contain medications for symptoms you don't have, and therefore may result in needless overtreatment. Avoid them entirely for children under 13; even those cold preparations marketed especially for children don't seem to work for this age group, and the drugs commonly induce drowsiness, making everything worse. Over-the-counter decongestants can help break up nasal congestion, but only temporarily: If these drugs are taken regularly for more than five days, your body may rebound from them and produce even more mucus—and worse congestion. Pseudoephedrine, one decongestant, increases blood pressure and heart rate; do not take it without first checking with your doctor if you have heart disease, high blood pressure, prostate problems, diabetes, or thyroid problems.

Over-the-counter cough suppressants, such as those containing dextromethorphan, can be helpful if your cough is so severe that it interferes with sleeping or talking. Otherwise, allow yourself to cough as you need to (always covering your mouth as you do), because coughing

C A U T I O N !

Never give aspirin to a child with a fever; give paracetamol instead. Reye's syndrome, a neurological disease that can cause coma, brain damage, and death, has been linked to aspirin use in children aged 4 to 15. Reye's syndrome is rare, but typically follows a viral infection: One to three days after the virus has set in, the child becomes extremely tired, vomits heavily, and may be agitated, delirious, and/or confused. Reye's syndrome is an emergency that requires urgent intravenous fluid replacement.

removes mucus and germs from your throat and lungs. Over-the-counter antihistamines can temporarily make breathing easier, but at a cost: They clear the nose by drying it up, making nasal mucus thicker and harder to drain.

COMPLEMENTARY CHOICES

Time and rest are of the essence: Begin to treat your cold as soon as you feel the first symptom. Especially with herbal remedies, an early response often results in a faster and more comfortable recovery.

AROMATHERAPY

Herbal steam can reduce congestion, and if the vapour temperature is over 43°C, it will also kill cold germs on contact. Choose eucalyptus *(Eucalyptus globulus)*, wintergreen *(Gaultheria procumbens)*, or peppermint *(Mentha piperita)*. Place either fresh leaves or a few drops of the herb's oil in a bowl and pour in boiling water. Place a towel over your head, lean over the bowl to create a steam tent, and breathe the vapour.

HERBAL THERAPIES

Taken at the first sign of symptoms, echinacea *(Echinacea* spp.) can reduce a cold's intensity and duration, often even preventing it from becoming a full-fledged infection. Echinacea apparently stimulates the immune response, enhancing resistance to all infection. It is available in capsules or tea: Add 2 tsp echinacea root to 1 cup water; simmer for 15 minutes and drink three cups daily. Goldenseal *(Hydrastis canadensis)* helps clear mucus from the throat. It also contains the natural antibiotic berberine, which can help prevent bacterial infections that often follow colds. Steep ½ to 1 tsp goldenseal in 1 cup boiling water for 10 to 15 minutes; drink three cups daily.

For a good 'cold tea', combine equal parts of elder *(Sambucus nigra)*, peppermint *(Mentha piperita)*, and yarrow *(Achillea millefolium)* and steep 1 to 2 tsp of the mixture in 1 cup hot water. This blend can help the body handle fever and reduce aches, congestion, and inflammation.

Garlic *(Allium sativum)* appears to shorten a cold's duration and severity. Any form seems to work: capsules or tablets, oil rubbed on the skin, or whole garlic roasted or cooked in other foods. If you elect capsules, take 3, three times daily, until the cold is over.

HOMEOPATHY

Cold symptoms often respond well to homeopathic remedies. The dosage is 12c, taken every two hours for a maximum of four doses. Gelsemium may help if you have chills, aching arms and legs, and fatigue, or if your throat hurts. When your runny nose feels as though it burns, your eyes water constantly, and you sneeze often, try Allium cepa. If you feel irritable and have a runny nose that becomes congested at night, take Nux vomica. For a barking cough, a burning sore throat, and a bitter taste that lingers in your mouth, try Aconite.

LIFESTYLE

Refrain from smoking, especially when you have a cold. Smoking assaults the mucous membranes and lungs, increasing your susceptibility to all sorts of respiratory infections, including colds. Once you have a cold, smoke irritates the already-inflamed tissues, making healing and recovery more difficult.

NUTRITION AND DIET

Good nutrition is essential for resisting and recovering from a cold. Eat a balanced diet. Take supplements as needed to ensure you are receiving the recommended dietary allowances for vitamin A, the vitamin B complex (vitamins B_1, B_2, B_5, B_6, folic acid), and vitamin C, as well as the minerals zinc and copper. If your diet is deficient in zinc, your body is low in white blood cells, and you're an easy target for all types of infections, including colds. Zinc is available as a tablet or throat lozenge.

While you have a cold, avoid dairy products, which tend to make mucus thicker.

The last 20 years have witnessed much research into whether or not taking megadoses (1 gram or more each day) of vitamin C will prevent colds. Results have varied, but it appears that megadoses of vitamin C cannot prevent colds.

Chicken soup has been heralded as a cold

therapy since the 12th century. Recent scientific evidence supports the notion that chicken soup reduces cold symptoms, especially congestion. Something (yet to be determined) in the chicken soup keeps white blood cells from clumping together and causing inflammation.

Any food spicy enough to make your eyes water will have the same effect on your nose, promoting drainage. If you feel like eating, a hot, spicy choice will help your body fight your cold.

HOME REMEDIES

◆ Research shows that if you
◆ Suck cough sweets to soothe your sore throat, but stay away from mint varieties as they can be drying.
◆ Dab petroleum jelly in and around your nostrils to protect against chafing.
◆ Keep your body hydrated by drinking at least 10 glasses of water each day; this will replace the fluids lost through perspiration and your runny nose and minimize nasal and chest congestion. Keep a glass of water on your bedside table to sip during the night.
◆ Humidify your room (especially during the colder months when central heating dries the air) to keep the mucous membranes of your nose and throat moist.

PREVENTION

A strong immune system is the best defence against all infections, colds included. Boost your body's natural resistance by eating well, not smoking, and drinking plenty of water every day. Minimize contact with people who have colds, or at the very least don't share towels, cutlery, or beverages with them. Cold viruses often survive for hours in the open, on doorknobs, money, and other surfaces, so wash your hands frequently.

When you have a cold, do your best to keep it to yourself and, if possible, stay at home for the first two days. A hearty sneeze can carry your cold virus up to 4 metres away, so always cover your mouth when you sneeze (or cough).

Regular, moderate exercise (such as walking for 45 minutes, five times a week) appears to strengthen the immune system and make you less likely to get colds and other infections. Saunas may also help: Swedish researchers have evidence that taking at least two saunas each week can keep you from succumbing to a cold. The reason is unclear, although the sauna's heat may prevent cold germs from reproducing. ■

CONJUNCTIVITIS

- Burning itchy eyes that discharge a heavy, sticky mucus may indicate **bacterial conjunctivitis.**
- Copious tears, a swollen lymph node, and a light discharge of mucus from one eye are signs of **viral conjunctivitis.**
- Redness, intense itching, and tears in the eyes may indicate **allergic conjunctivitis.**

CALL YOUR DOCTOR IF:

- you physically injure your eye. Eye injuries can become infected and lead to corneal ulcers, which can endanger your eyesight.
- your eyes become red when you wear contact lenses. Remove the lenses immediately and see your ophthalmologist; you may have a corneal infection.
- the redness in your eye is affecting your vision and is accompanied by severe pain or excessive yellow or green discharge. You may have a staphylococcal infection or a streptococcal infection.
- your conjunctivitis frequently recurs or appears to be getting worse after a week of home treatment; you may have a bacterial or viral infection.
- your newborn baby's eyes are inflamed and are not producing tears; this may indicate **ophthalmia neonatorum,** which must be treated immediately to prevent permanent eye damage.

The conjunctiva—the transparent membrane that lines your eyeball and your eyelid—can become inflamed for various reasons. Most cases of conjunctivitis run a predictable course, and the inflammation usually clears up in a few days. Although conjunctivitis can be highly contagious, it is rarely serious and will not damage your vision if detected and treated promptly.

Bacterial conjunctivitis, commonly known as **pinkeye,** usually infects both eyes and produces a heavy discharge of mucus.

Viral conjunctivitis is usually limited to one eye, causing copious tears and a light discharge.

Allergic conjunctivitis produces tears, itching, and redness in the eyes, and sometimes an itchy, runny nose.

Ophthalmia neonatorum is an acute form of **inclusion conjunctivitis** in newborn babies. It must be treated immediately by a hospital specialist to prevent permanent eye damage or blindness.

CAUSES

Conjunctivitis is caused by a bacterial or viral infection or by an allergic reaction to pollen, smoke, or other material that irritates your eyes. Children sometimes contract conjunctivitis after a cold or sore throat. Redness and inflammation of the conjunctiva can also be brought on by eyestrain, stress, and poor nutrient levels.

Ophthalmia neonatorum may occur if the baby's tear ducts are not completely opened or if the infant is exposed to bacteria when passing through the birth canal of a mother infected with chlamydia or gonorrhoea. The herpes virus may also be associated with conjunctivitis and corneal infection.

TREATMENT

Traditionally, home remedies have been sufficient for soothing conjunctivitis associated with uncomplicated colds, minor infections, or allergies. Treatment consists primarily of cleansing the eyes and preventing the condition from spreading.

The conjunctiva is a thin, protective membrane that covers the exposed white of the eye and the inside of the eyelid. Bacterial conjunctivitis—sometimes called pinkeye—is the result of an infection that makes the conjunctiva red, teary, and itchy, with a thick, greenish yellow discharge. When conjunctivitis is caused by an allergy, the discharge may be clear and watery or yellowish.

Eyelid, Conjunctiva, Cornea, Lens

CONVENTIONAL MEDICINE

If your conjunctivitis symptoms do not appear to be associated with a cold or allergy, you may want to see your doctor or an ophthalmologist for a medical diagnosis. For **bacterial conjunctivitis,** the treatment will probably call for antibiotic eye drops or ointment. **Allergic conjunctivitis** may respond to antihistamine or steroid eye drops, but you should not use steroid drops for either **bacterial** or **viral conjunctivitis.**

COMPLEMENTARY CHOICES

Complementary therapies rely on natural remedies to soothe your irritated eyes and ease the itching and inflammation.

HERBAL THERAPIES

Using an eyecup, wash the eye several times a day with one of the following solutions. In each case, cool and strain the eyewash before using.
◆ 1 tsp dried eyebright (*Euphrasia rostkoviana*)

steeped in half a litre of boiling water.
◆ 2 to 3 tsp chamomile (*Chamaemelum nobile*) in half a litre of boiling water.

HOMEOPATHY

Depending on your symptoms, take the following remedies four times daily for one or two days:
◆ for stinging eyes and red, puffy eyelids, Apis 12x.
◆ for bloodshot eyes and a gritty feeling, Argentum nitricum 12x.
◆ for itchy eyes with a sticky, yellow discharge, Pulsatilla 12x.

HOME REMEDIES

You can cleanse and soothe irritated eyes with a prepared boric acid eyewash, or try the herbal eyewashes above. To relieve discomfort of **bacterial** or **viral conjunctivitis,** apply a warm compress for 5 to 10 minutes, three to four times a day. For **allergic conjunctivitis,** place a cool compress or a cool, moist tea bag on your closed eye. If the condition does not improve in five days, consult an ophthalmologist.

PREVENTION

Bacterial and **viral conjunctivitis** are highly contagious. Unless you take preventive measures, the condition may spread to your other eye and to other people.
◆ Wash your hands often and well.
◆ Keep your hands away from the infected eye.
◆ Do not share washcloths, towels, pillowcases, or handkerchiefs with other family members.
◆ Change your washcloth, towel, and pillowcase after each use, and wash them thoroughly.
◆ Do not use other people's eye cosmetics, particularly eye pencils and mascara.
If your child gets **pinkeye,** keep him or her out of school for a few days. Once one student comes down with conjunctivitis, it is not uncommon for it to spread to an entire class. ■

SYMPTOMS

- a sharp, barking cough, usually accompanied by trouble inhaling and sometimes by a hoarse voice caused by inflamed vocal cords.
- laboured breathing that seems to put strain on the neck muscles, ribs, or breastbone, making these areas retract noticeably with each breath.

CALL YOUR DOCTOR IF:

- your child has croup accompanied by a high fever (39°C or more).
- home remedies are not working and the croup symptoms seem to be worsening; hospitalization may be required.
- your child has croup and his respiratory rate is fast, he is having extreme difficulty in breathing, he cannot talk, or he is turning pale or blue. These are all symptoms of severe respiratory distress. **Call 999 for immediate emergency help.**
- your child is younger than the age of five and has noisy, rapid breathing; a foreign object may be stuck in his throat.
- your child suddenly begins drooling or can't swallow, has a high fever but no cough, and is leaning forward but can't bend his neck and can't talk. Your child may have a dangerous bacterial infection called epiglottitis, which causes a blocked airway. Do not open the mouth to look inside; doing so can completely close the throat and shut down the child's breathing. **Call 999 for immediate emergency help.**

Croup, a viral infection of the voice box (larynx) associated with signs of a respiratory infection, such as a runny nose or cough, is a relatively common ailment of childhood. Usually the first indication is a cough that sounds like the bark of a seal. Your child may have trouble breathing because the tissue around the larynx is inflamed, constricting the windpipe, and because the bronchial passages are blocked with mucus. The sound of air being forced through the narrowed airways may produce hollow raspy noises with each inhaled breath.

Croup lasts for five or six days and is highly contagious. It usually affects children between three months and six years old (the average age is two), whose small windpipes and bronchial passages are vulnerable to blockage. Most cases are mild and can be managed at home. In severe cases or in the case of epiglottitis—an unrelated bacterial infection of the epiglottis (the flap covering the trachea), whose symptoms mimic croup—your child may need to be hospitalized.

CAUSES

Most croup cases are caused by a para-influenza virus. The disease is transmitted by airborne droplets from an infected child's cough.

TREATMENT

You and your child may be panicked by the apparent sudden onset of a croup attack. Try to

WARNING!

If your child can't breathe, cough, or speak and he is leaning forward with his neck thrust out, do not open his mouth or tilt his head back to look inside. His throat could close completely, causing respiratory arrest. Call 999. If your child stops breathing, begin CPR immediately (see Cardiac and Respiratory Arrest).

ACUPRESSURE

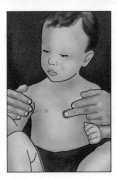 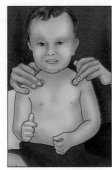

1 Gentle pressure on Conception Vessel 17 may help to calm a baby suffering from croup. Place your finger in the centre of the child's chest, midway between the nipples, and press lightly. Hold for one minute and release.

2 Coughing spasms may be eased by pressure on Lung 1. Place one finger of each hand about 1 centimetre below the large hollow under the collarbone, on the outer part of the chest near the shoulder. Apply pressure gently for one minute.

keep your child calm; crying will only make breathing more difficult. Croup usually can be managed with mist or steam therapy, which dissolves sticky or dried mucus in the child's breathing passages. Because the condition commonly worsens at night, many doctors recommend that you sleep in the same room with your child or use a baby-monitoring device to listen for any change in the child's condition. Be ready to get emergency medical help if your child doesn't improve.

CONVENTIONAL MEDICINE

Doctors recommend home care for all but the most serious cases of croup. If the symptoms are severe enough, your pediatrician may take x-rays to check for epiglottitis—which would be treated with antibiotics during a short hospital stay. Severe cases of croup may also require hospitalization; the child will be given inhaled medications such as adrenaline or oral corticosteroids to counter swelling.

COMPLEMENTARY CHOICES

ACUPRESSURE

Practitioners suggest pressing at least four of the following points in succession: Large Intestine 4; Triple Warmer 5; Bladder 12, 13; Lung 1, 2; Conception Vessel 17; and Governing Vessel 24. *(See pages 138-139 for information on point locations.)*

HERBAL THERAPIES

To alleviate a persistent cough, herbalists use aniseed *(Pimpinella anisum),* sundew *(Drosera rotundifolia),* or thyme *(Thymus vulgaris),* which are said to act as mild cough suppressants.

HOMEOPATHY

Aconite, favored by homeopaths for croup, can be given in the 12x or 30c dosage at the beginning of an attack and then every 30 minutes until the child can sleep. If Aconite doesn't work or if the child's breathing sounds like wood being sawed, try Spongia in the same dosage and intervals. For a more mucus-filled bronchial cough, Hepar sulphuris is the third choice for acute croup.

HOME REMEDIES

◆ A cool-mist humidifier may help your child breathe. Direct the mist away from the face and don't put medications in the water; they may irritate your child's throat.
◆ Steam may help loosen phlegm and relax the throat. Turn on the shower and let steam accumulate in your bathroom. Carry your child around in the room (but not under the shower) until the child's breathing becomes easier.
◆ Cold air sometimes offsets croup. If the night is cool, take your child for a ride in the car with the windows down.
◆ Paracetamol will bring down a fever and lower your child's respiratory rate.
◆ Offer plenty of non-citric liquids to restore fluids and to loosen phlegm.
◆ Keep your child away from cigarette smoke.■

EARACHE

Read down this column to find your symptoms. Then read across.

SYMPTOMS	AILMENT/PROBLEM
◆ earache that gets worse over weeks or months; blocked feeling and ringing in the ears; partial hearing loss.	◆ Excess earwax that has hardened in the outer ear canal, blocking the eardrum
◆ following air travel or scuba diving, ear pain that may radiate into the cheeks and forehead; dizziness; ringing in the ears; ears feel blocked.	◆ Barotrauma (strained or damaged eardrum, due to large changes in atmospheric pressure)
◆ feeling that something is in your ear; hearing loss; ear pain.	◆ Presence of a foreign object, such as a bug, a seed, or an earplug, in the ear
◆ itching in the ear, later becoming sharp or dull ear pain; pain worsens if you pull on your earlobe; yellowish discharge; possibly, fever and temporary hearing loss.	◆ Swimmer's ear
◆ ear pain that is either sharp and sudden or dull and throbbing; fever; nasal congestion; muffled hearing.	◆ Otitis media
◆ pressure in the ear; a lump outside or inside the ear canal; excessive earwax; possibly, hearing loss and infection (fever, ear pain, and swelling).	◆ A benign (non-cancerous) cyst or tumour in or just outside the ear canal
◆ earache; persistent tooth or jaw pain.	◆ Tooth or gum trouble, such as tooth decay or abscess; temporomandibular joint syndrome
◆ dull pain, redness, and swelling both within and behind the ear; mild fever; thick pus discharge from ear; possibly, partial hearing loss.	◆ Mastoiditis (infection of the mastoid process, the honeycomb-like bone behind the ear)
◆ sudden ear pain, usually after an injury or an infection; bleeding or pus discharge from the ear; dizziness; ringing in the ear; partial hearing loss.	◆ Ruptured eardrum

- For three days, place a few drops of warm baby oil or almond or olive oil in the ear twice daily to soften wax. Then use a bulb syringe to flush out the wax with warm water.

- Flushing the ear may cause dizziness. Never try to remove wax by inserting an object—even a cotton wool bud—in your ear; you could damage your eardrum and your hair.

- Symptoms should dissipate within a few hours without treatment. If they don't, consult your doctor.

- During flight, hold your nose and gently blow air into it, or constantly suck a boiled sweet or chew gum; this may help equalize the pressure on either side of your eardrum.

- See Emergencies/First Aid: Ear Emergencies.

- Never try to remove an object that is lodged in your ear; you risk perforating your eardrum. See your doctor.

- Take paracetamol for pain. Your doctor may also prescribe ear drops containing an antibiotic, an antifungal drug, or cortisone (to reduce inflammation).

- Keep water out of your ears (when swimming and showering) for at least three weeks after symptoms have subsided. Don't use earplugs; they can be harmful.

- Place a warm compress over the ear and take paracetamol. Call your doctor; you may need prescription antibiotics.

- A few drops of warm mineral or olive oil in your ear may lessen pain.

- Often no treatment is needed. If the cyst or tumour becomes extremely large or infected, your doctor will remove it.

- Call your dentist today. An abscessed tooth is an emergency. See also Toothache.

- Relaxation techniques may ease mild cases of temporomandibular joint syndrome.

- Call your doctor today. You need aggressive antibiotic therapy, perhaps for several weeks. Persistent infection may call for surgical removal of the mastoid process.

- Without treatment, mastoiditis can cause serious problems, such as meningitis and facial paralysis.

- Take paracetamol for pain until you can see a doctor. You may need a patch for the eardrum (to speed healing) and antibiotics. Large tears can be surgically repaired.

- Don't blow your nose or allow water in your ear until the rupture has healed (which should take two months or so).

FLU

SYMPTOMS

- fever—usually around 38°C, but occasionally as high as 41°C—sometimes alternating with chills.
- sore throat.
- dry, hacking cough.
- aching muscles.
- general fatigue and weakness.
- nasal congestion, sneezing.
- headache.

CALL YOUR DOCTOR IF:

- you experience any of these symptoms and your immune system is already weakened by cancer, diabetes, AIDS, or other conditions; or if you have a serious illness such as chronic heart or kidney disease, impaired breathing, cystic fibrosis, or chronic anaemia. You may be at risk of developing serious secondary complications and need to be carefully monitored as long as symptoms last.
- your fever lasts more than three or four days, you become short of breath while resting, or you have chest pain. You may have developed bronchitis, pleurisy or pneumonia.

Influenza—commonly shortened to 'flu'—is an extremely contagious viral disease that appears most frequently in winter and early spring. The infection spreads through your upper respiratory tract and sometimes goes into your lungs. The virus typically sweeps through large groups of people who share indoor space, such as schools, offices, and nursing homes. Worldwide, influenza has killed many millions of people.

Although both colds and influenza stem from viruses that infect the upper respiratory tract, the symptoms of influenza are more pronounced and its complications more severe. Influenza occurs most commonly in school-age children, but its most severe effects are felt by infants, the elderly, and people with chronic ailments. Despite advances in prevention and treatment, influenza and its complications are still fatal to thousands of people every year. Specific strains of the disease can be prevented by injections of antibodies in a flu vaccine, but after influenza—or any other viral infection, for that matter—has started, there is no cure except to let it run its course.

CAUSES

The flu virus is transmitted by inhaling droplets in the air that contain the virus, or by handling items contaminated by an infected person. The symptoms start to develop from one to four days after infection with the virus.

Researchers divide influenza viruses into three general categories: types A, B, and C. While all three types can mutate, or change into new strains, type A influenza mutates constantly, yielding new strains of the virus every few years. This means that you can never develop a permanent immunity to influenza. Even if you develop antibodies against a flu virus one year, those antibodies are unlikely to protect you against a new strain of the virus the next year. Type A mutations are responsible for major epidemics every several years. Types B and C are less common and result in local outbreaks and milder cases. Type B has also been linked to the development of Reye's syndrome, a potentially fatal complication of influenza and other viral infections—such as chickenpox—that usually affect children.

Most influenza viruses that infect humans seem to originate in parts of Asia where close contact between livestock and people creates a hospitable environment for the mutation and transmission of viruses. Swine, or pigs, can catch both avian (meaning from birds or poultry) and human forms of a virus, and act as hosts for these different viral strains to meet and mutate into new forms. The swine then infect people with the new form of the virus in the same way in which people infect each other—by transmitting viruses through the exchange of droplets in the air.

DIAGNOSTIC AND TEST PROCEDURES

All three types of influenza mimic the basic symptoms of the common cold, such as cough and headache. Your doctor may take a throat culture or blood test to rule out the possibility of other ailments such as streptococcal throat or, if public-health officials are gathering statistics on an influenza outbreak, to identify the specific viral strain.

TREATMENT

Influenza will run its course regardless of how you treat it. Because it is a viral disease, it does not respond to antibiotics. If you are in good health, influenza will probably pass with no complications after a week or so of bed rest and self-care at home. If you are over 65, are a diabetic, or have another chronic disease, talk to your doctor about being immunized before winter sets in (see Prevention, page 91). If you then come down with flu anyway, make sure your doctor monitors your progress so that any complications can be caught and treated appropriately.

CONVENTIONAL MEDICINE

Doctors have no single treatment that applies to all cases of influenza. You will probably be told to rest in bed, eat nourishing food, and drink lots of liquids. Fluids are especially important to help avoid dehydration from fever and for loosening up respiratory tract secretions.

You can try over-the-counter medicines to ease the discomfort of your cough, nasal congestion, and sore throat. A steam vaporizer in your room puts moisture into the air and may make breathing easier. If you are feverish and have muscle aches, analgesics like aspirin, ibuprofen, or paracetamol may help you feel better. Because aspirin has been linked to Reye's syndrome, you should not give it to children.

If these remedies don't help a severe bout of flu, your doctor may give you oral antiviral drugs that are active against type A influenza. You need to give yourself time to fully recuperate from influenza and prevent the development of secondary infections that can cause bronchitis, sinusitis, or pneumonia.

A COLD OR THE FLU: WHICH IS IT?

The common cold and influenza are both contagious viral infections of the respiratory tract. Although the symptoms can be similar, influenza is worse: A cold may drag you down a bit, but influenza can make you shudder at the very thought of getting out of bed.

Congestion, sore throat, and sneezing are common with colds, and both ailments bring coughing, headache, and chest discomfort. With influenza you are likely to run a high fever for several days, and your head and body will ache. Usually, complications from colds are relatively minor, but a severe case of influenza can lead to a life-threatening illness like pneumonia.

Over 200 types of cold viruses are known, and new strains of influenza evolve every few years. Since both diseases are viral, neither can be conquered by antibiotics; those drugs are useful only against a secondary bacterial infection that may cause sinusitis or pneumonia.

COMPLEMENTARY CHOICES

Complementary therapies may help strengthen your body's ability to fight the virus and recover from the illness as well as ease temporary flu symptoms.

ACUPRESSURE

Pressure on a number of points can be recommended for various flu symptoms; refer to pages 8-9 for the location of acupressure points. Bladder 36 is recommended for stimulating natural resistance to colds and flu. Bladder 2, Stomach 3, Large Intestine 20, Gall Bladder 20, and Governing Vessels 16 and 24 may be helpful for relieving nasal congestion, headaches, and eyestrain. Large Intestine 11 may help fight fever and strengthen your immune system. Large Intestine 4 may offer general relief from flu symptoms, but do not press it if you are pregnant. Conception Vessel 22 and Kidney 27 may help relieve chest congestion and coughing. Finally, try Bladder 38 to relieve coughing, breathing difficulties, and other respiratory complications.

AROMATHERAPY

In flu season, when those around you are coming down with the virus, protect yourself by gargling daily with one drop each of the essential oils of tea tree (*Melaleuca* spp.) and lemon in a glass of warm water; stir well before each mouthful. If you come down with the flu despite your best preventive measures, 2 drops of tea tree oil in a hot bath may help your immune system fight the viral infection and ease your symptoms. Tea tree oil can be irritating to the skin, however, so don't use more than 2 drops in a full bath.

If you have a congested nose or chest, add a few drops of essential oils of eucalyptus (*Eucalyptus globulus*) or peppermint (*Mentha piperita*) to a steam vaporizer. If you are asthmatic, do not use steam; instead, sprinkle a few drops of these essential oils on a handkerchief and inhale.

HERBAL THERAPIES

For an herbal approach to stimulating your immune system, try taking ½ tsp each of tincture of goldenseal (*Hydrastis canadensis*) and echinacea (*Echinacea* spp.) twice a day. If flu symptoms appear, chew a clove of raw garlic (*Allium sativum*) for its antiviral properties, but do not eat raw garlic on an empty stomach.

An infusion of boneset (*Eupatorium perfoliatum*) may relieve aches and fever and clear congestion: Simmer 1 cup boiling water with 2 tsp of the herb for 10 to 15 minutes; drink a cupful every hour, as hot as you can stand it. To combat chills, try taking 30 drops of yarrow (*Achillea millefolium*) or elder (*Sambucus nigra*) flower tincture every four hours until your chills are gone.

HOMEOPATHY

For homeopathic self-care, try one of the following remedies in 12c dosages every 6 to 8 hours for a day or two. If you don't notice an improvement in your condition after 24 hours, try another homeopathic remedy.

◆ If you feel tired, weak, 'heavy', and chilled, with headache and stuffy nose, try Gelsemium.
◆ If you feel general aching in your muscles, with headache and irritability that are worse when you move around, and if you are thirsty for cold fluids and have a dry hacking cough, try Bryonia.
◆ If you are restless, chilled, and thirsty with a dry mouth, hoarse voice, and aching joints, try Rhus toxicodendron.
◆ If you have a dry cough and generalized aches, or if your body feels bruised and chilled, and you are thirsty for cold drinks although they upset your stomach, try Eupatorium perfoliatum.

NUTRITION AND DIET

Eat vitamin C-rich fresh fruits and vegetables like citrus fruits, Brussels sprouts, and strawberries; and take up to 100 mg per day of vitamin C. Increase zinc intake with lean meats, fish, and whole-grain breads and cereals.

REFLEXOLOGY

To support your respiratory system, press your thumb into the solar plexus/diaphragm point for a few seconds, or massage the point with your thumb.

HOME REMEDIES

◆ Take two tablets of aspirin, paracetamol, or ibuprofen every four hours to reduce fever, headache, and body aches: These symptoms are usually worst in the afternoon and evening. Do not give aspirin to anyone under 12, because some people in this age group may be at risk of developing Reye's syndrome.

◆ If you have a sore or scratchy throat, try a salt-water gargle. Dissolve 1 tsp salt in half a litre of warm water. Gargle whenever your throat is uncomfortable, but don't swallow the mixture.

◆ Use a heating pad on body aches.

◆ When you feel like eating, try soups and bland, starchy food like dry toast, bananas, apple sauce, cottage cheese, boiled rice, rice pudding, cooked cereal, and baked potatoes. These foods provide a gentle transition for your digestive system when you have not been eating regularly.

◆ Don't drink alcoholic beverages; they leave you dehydrated and can lower your body's ability to fight illness and secondary infection. Avoid over-the-counter flu remedies that contain alcohol.

◆ If you take over-the-counter pain relievers, make sure your symptoms are actually diminishing, not just temporarily suppressed, before you get out of bed. If you don't give yourself enough time to recover fully, you may end up prolonging your illness or developing debilitating complications.

PREVENTION

The most effective preventive measure against influenza is to be inoculated every autumn against strains that have developed since the previous outbreak. If you are vaccinated against one or more type A and B strains, you may still come down with flu, but your symptoms are likely to be milder than they would have been had you not had a vaccination.

Influenza vaccine is available through your GP and public-health facilities. Because influenza is a serious threat, the vaccination is recommended for everyone over 65; nursing home residents and employees; anyone whose immune system is compromised by AIDS, cancer, or other chronic ailments; anyone who suffers from chronic bronchitis; and people who work in medical facilities. The vaccine is usually given as a single injection, although children may receive two. If you are pregnant, wait until your second trimester and make sure your doctor approves of the vaccination. Some people develop low fever and muscle aches as side effects of the vaccine. Because the vaccine is grown in chicken embryos, it is not recommended for people who are allergic to eggs.

Oral antiviral medications may lessen your risk of contracting type A flu, but they are most effective if you begin to take them a few weeks before the flu season begins or within two days after symptoms appear. Usually these drugs are prescribed for people at high risk for developing complications from flu, such as people with chronic lung disease or the elderly. If the virus has already begun to circulate in your community, a doctor may also prescribe medication while you are waiting for a vaccination. If so, continue taking it for two weeks after you are vaccinated to ensure that you are adequately protected while your body builds up its immune response to the vaccine. Other preventive measures you can take during flu season are to:

◆ Give up smoking—which damages your respiratory tract—and alcohol, since both substances lower your resistance to infection in general.

◆ Avoid sleeping in a room with someone who has flu; the virus is easily spread in the air.

◆ Wash your hands often to kill viruses you may have picked up by touching contaminated objects like doorknobs or phone receivers.

◆ Try to avoid crowds, and give people who are coughing or sneezing a wide berth. Aeroplanes are especially effective at exposing people to flu viruses because cabin air is recirculated.

◆ Stay warm and dry so that your body can fight off infection by flu and other viruses. ■

- bright red anal bleeding that may streak the bowel movement or the toilet tissue.
- tenderness or pain during bowel movements.
- painful swelling or a lump near the anus.
- anal itching.
- a mucous anal discharge.

CALL YOUR DOCTOR IF:

- you experience any anal bleeding for the first time, even if you believe you have haemorrhoids. Colon polyps, colitis, Crohn's disease, and colorectal cancer can also cause anal bleeding. An accurate diagnosis is essential.
- you have been diagnosed with hemorrhoids, and you have anal bleeding that is chronic (daily or weekly) or more profuse than the streaking described above. Though rare, excessive haemorrhoidal bleeding can cause anemia.

Haemorrhoids are essentially varicose veins of the rectum. The haemorrhoidal veins are located in the lowest area of the rectum and the anus. Sometimes they swell, so that the vein walls become stretched, thin, and irritated by passing bowel movements. When these swollen veins bleed, itch, or hurt, they are known as haemorrhoids, or piles. Haemorrhoids are classified into two general categories: internal and external.

Internal haemorrhoids lie far enough inside the rectum that you can't see or feel them. They don't usually hurt, because there are few pain-sensing nerves in the rectum. Bleeding may be the only sign of their presence. Sometimes internal haemorrhoids prolapse, or enlarge and protrude outside the anal sphincter. If so, you may be able to see or feel them as moist, pink pads of skin that are pinker than the surrounding area. Prolapsed haemorrhoids may hurt, because the anus is dense with pain-sensing nerves. They usually recede into the rectum on their own; if they don't, they can be gently pushed back into place.

External hemorrhoids lie within the anus and are usually painful. If an external haemorrhoid prolapses to the outside (usually in the course of passing a stool) you can see and feel it. Blood clots sometimes form within prolapsed external haemorrhoids, causing an extremely painful condition called a thrombosis. If an external haemorrhoid becomes thrombosed, it can look rather frightening, turning purple or blue, and possibly bleeding. Despite their appearance, thrombosed haemorrhoids are usually not serious and will resolve themselves in about a week. If the pain is unbearable, a doctor can remove the thrombosis, which stops the pain, during a surgery or hospital visit.

Anal bleeding and pain of any sort is alarming and should be evaluated; it can indicate a life-threatening condition, such as colorectal cancer. Haemorrhoids are the most common cause of anal bleeding and are rarely dangerous but a definite diagnosis from your physician is a must.

CAUSES

About half of us will suffer from haemorrhoids at

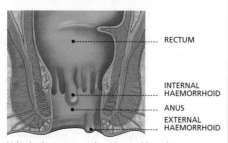

WHERE HAEMORRHOIDS FORM

RECTUM

INTERNAL HAEMORRHOID

ANUS

EXTERNAL HAEMORRHOID

Veins in the rectum and anus are subjected to considerable pressure whenever a stool is passed. Pushing or straining may cause veins in the rectal wall to bulge, creating clusters of swollen, or dilated, veins called haemorrhoids. Internal haemorrhoids can form anywhere inside the anal canal, while external haemorrhoids are visible at, or just below, the opening of the anus.

some point in life; for most, this will happen between ages 20 and 50. Researchers are not certain what causes haemorrhoids. 'Weak' veins—leading to haemorrhoids and other varicose veins—may be inherited. It's likely that extreme abdominal pressure causes the veins to swell and become susceptible to irritation. Sources of this pressure include obesity, pregnancy, standing or sitting for long periods, liver disease, straining from constipation or diarrhoea, coughing, sneezing, vomiting, and holding one's breath while straining to do physical labour.

Diet has a pivotal role in causing—and preventing—haemorrhoids. People who consistently eat a high-fibre diet are unlikely to get haemorrhoids, whereas those who prefer a diet high in refined foods can expect them. A low-fibre diet or inadequate fluid intake causes constipation, which contributes to haemorrhoids in two ways: It encourages straining to have a bowel movement, and it also aggravates the hemorrhoids by producing hard stools that further irritate the swollen veins.

DIAGNOSTIC AND TEST PROCEDURES

Your doctor will first visually examine the anal

area, perhaps by inserting a lubricated gloved finger or an anoscope (a hollow, lighted tube for viewing the lower few centimetres of the rectum) or a proctoscope (which works like an anoscope but provides a more thorough rectal examination). More procedures may be needed to identify internal haemorrhoids or rule out other ailments that frequently cause anal bleeding, such as anal fissure, colitis, Crohn's disease, and colorectal cancer. To see further into the anal canal (into the lower colon, or sigmoid), sigmoidoscopy may be used, or the entire colon may be viewed with colonoscopy. For both procedures, a lighted, flexible viewing tube is inserted into the rectum. A barium x-ray can show the entire colon's interior. First a barium enema is given, then x-rays are taken of the lower gastrointestinal tract.

TREATMENT

Once you have them, haemorrhoids don't usually go away completely unless you undergo one of the procedures below. They can get better, however, so that living with them is tolerable. Both conventional and complementary practitioners consider diet the best tool for treating haemorrhoids. A diet rich in high-fibre foods and low in refined and junk foods is essential. Probably half of all haemorrhoid sufferers find relief with dietary changes alone.

Most haemorrhoid treatments aim to minimize pain and itching. Warm (but not hot) sitz baths are the most time-honoured and often suggested therapy: Sit in about 8cm of warm water for 15 minutes, several times a day, especially after a bowel movement. If you are pregnant, discuss any treatment, including dietary changes, with your doctor before proceeding.

CONVENTIONAL MEDICINE

If you have been diagnosed as having haemorrhoids, a high-fibre diet combined with sitz baths and paracetamol should reduce discomfort within two weeks. If symptoms persist, your physician may suggest one of the following procedures. All except laser coagulation and surgery can be performed at hospital outpatients'.

Injection. An internal haemorrhoid can be injected with phenol in oil, quinine, and urea, or morrhuate sodium, which creates a scar and closes off the haemorrhoid. The injection hurts only a little, as any injection does. With a success rate of 90 per cent, this is many physicians' first choice. Results are not permanent, however; repeat injections may be needed every two or three years.

OVER-THE-COUNTER RELIEF

Controversy continues to rage about the efficacy of hemorrhoid medicines. We annually spend thousands of pounds on creams, ointments, and suppositories that promise to relieve inflammation and pain.

The basic ingredient in all these medicines is a lubricant, such as lanolin, cocoa butter, vegetable oil, or one of many others. Some also include an anaesthetic such as benzocaine or lidocaine, or an astringent such as tannic acid or zinc compounds, purported to reduce swelling by constricting capillaries. Hemorrhoids, however, are not capillaries; they're veins, and astringents may have no effect on them. Anaesthetics may provide short-term relief, but only in cream or ointment form: Suppositories usually go too far up into the anal canal to help the hemorrhoids below.

Lubrication is the greatest benefit of most over-the-counter hemorrhoid medications. Plain petroleum jelly works as well and can be applied with your finger. For pain relief, try paracetamol and sitz baths.

Banding. Prolapsed haemorrhoids are often removed using rubber-band ligation. A special tool secures a tiny rubber band around the haemorrhoid, shutting off its blood supply almost instantly. Within a week, the haemorrhoid shrivels and falls off. This painless method is successful about 75 per cent of the time.

Coagulation or **cauterization.** Using either an electric probe, a laser beam, or an infrared light, a tiny burn painlessly seals the end of the haemorrhoid, causing it to close off and shrink. This is most useful for prolapsed haemorrhoids.

Surgery. For large internal haemorrhoids or extremely uncomfortable external haemorrhoids (such as thrombosed haemorrhoids that are too painful to live with), your consultant may elect traditional surgery, called haemorrhoidectomy. In the hospital, under general anaesthesia, the haemorrhoid is removed. After the operation, expect a week or so of bed rest, with analgesics prescribed for discomfort.

The success rate for haemorrhoid removal approaches 95 per cent, but unless dietary and lifestyle changes are made, haemorrhoids are likely to recur.

COMPLEMENTARY CHOICES

Try one or several of these therapies to alleviate haemorrhoid discomfort. If symptoms persist despite your efforts at relief, contact your doctor.

ACUPUNCTURE

The most responsive point for relieving haemorrhoid pain is Governing Vessel 20. Others that may augment it are Stomachs 25 and 36, Governing Vessel 14, and Large Intestine 11. See a licensed practitioner for treatment; see pages 138-139 for point locations.

HERBAL THERAPIES

Applied twice daily, pilewort *(Ranunculus ficaria)* ointment can reduce the pain of external hemorrhoids: Simmer 2 tbsp fresh or dried pilewort in 200 g petroleum jelly for 10 minutes. Allow to cool before using; store leftover ointment in a closed container. Pilewort may also be taken as a tea.

HOMEOPATHY

More than a dozen remedies, each taken at 12x, can help haemorrhoid pain. Choosing the right one requires attention to your symptoms and, usually, a homeopath's help. For a sore, bruised, and perhaps bleeding anus, try Hamamelis. Aesculus can ease sharp, spiking rectal pain that is worsened with bowel movements, and Sulphur can reduce burning and itching aggravated by warmth.

MASSAGE

This technique moves matter through the intestines, helping to prevent the constipation that contributes to haemorrhoids. Lie on your back, and use your fingers or your palm to make long, sweeping strokes. Repeat each stroke three to six times. Begin on your left side. Just below your ribs, stroke toward your feet; then stroke across your abdomen from the right to left just below your rib cage. Finally, point your fingertips toward your feet, and drag your hand up your right side from pelvis to ribs.

NUTRITION AND DIET

Prevent constipation by following a high-fibre diet. Meals and snacks should consist primarily of vegetables, fruit, nuts, and whole grains, and as few refined foods and meats as possible. If this is a big change for you, introduce the new foods slowly, to avoid wind. If you aren't able to eat enough high-fibre food, supplement your diet with psyllium stool softeners or bulk-forming agents. (Avoid laxatives, which cause diarrhoea that can further irritate the swollen veins.) Drink at least eight glasses of water each day; if your life is especially active or you live in a hot climate, you will need more. It's almost impossible to drink too much water.

Monitor your sodium intake. Excess salt in the diet causes fluid retention, which means swelling in all veins, including haemorrhoids.

HOME REMEDIES

◆ Try not to sit for hours at a time, but if you must, take breaks: Once every hour, get up and move around for at least five minutes. A doughnut-shaped cushion can make sitting more comfortable and ease haemorrhoid pressure and pain.

◆ Insert Vaseline petroleum jelly just inside the anus to make bowel movements less painful.

◆ Dab witch hazel (Hamamelis virginiana), a soothing anti-inflammatory agent, on irritated haemorrhoids to reduce pain and itching.

◆ Resist the temptation to scratch haemorrhoids, as it makes everything worse: The inflamed veins become more irritated, the skin around them becomes damaged, and the itching itself intensifies. Instead, to help stop the itching, apply an over-the-counter 0.5 percent hydrocortisone cream to the skin (not inside the anus—on the outside only) and a cold pack.

◆ If you need a pain reliever, try paracetamol. Avoid ibuprofen and aspirin, which may foster bleeding.

◆ Bathe regularly to keep the anal area clean, but be gentle: Excessive scrubbing, especially with soap, can intensify burning and irritation.

◆ Don't sit on the toilet for more than three minutes at a time, and when wiping, be gentle. If toilet paper is irritating, try dampening it first, or use cotton wool balls or alcohol-free baby wipes.

◆ When performing any task that requires exertion, be sure to breathe evenly. It's common to hold your breath during exertion, and if you do, you're straining, and contributing to haemorrhoid pain and bleeding.

PREVENTION

A healthy diet and lifestyle are good insurance for preventing haemorrhoids, whether you already suffer haemorrhoid symptoms or are intent on never experiencing them. Regular exercise is also important, especially if you work in a sedentary job. Exercise helps in several ways: keeping weight in check, making constipation less likely, and enhancing muscle tone which promotes the easy elimination of stools. ■

SYMPTOMS

If your headache is:

- a dull, steady pain that feels like a band tightening around your head, you have a **tension headache.**
- throbbing, begins on one side, and causes nausea, you have a **migraine.** Visual disturbances, such as flickering points of light, may precede the headache.
- a throbbing pain around one red, watery eye, with nasal congestion on that side of your face, you have a **cluster headache.**
- a steady pain in the area behind your face that gets worse if you bend forward and is accompanied by congestion, you have a **sinus headache.**

CALL YOUR DOCTOR IF:

- a severe headache is accompanied by vomiting, limb weakness, double vision, slurred speech, or difficulty in swallowing; you may have a cerebral hemorrhage or an aneurysm — **get medical help now.**
- your headache is of a kind you've never had, occurs first thing in the morning, is persistent, brings on vomiting, and abates during the day; you may have high blood pressure or in very rare cases a brain tumour. See your doctor without delay.
- you have a high fever, light hurts your eyes, the pain is severe and is accompanied by nausea and a stiff neck; you may have meningitis—**get medical help now.**
- after a head injury, you are drowsy, with dizziness, vertigo, nausea, or vomiting; you may have a concussion. See your doctor without delay.

Although painful and troublesome, most headaches are minor health concerns and can be easily treated with aspirin or another analgesic. But if they are severe, recur frequently, or are attended by other symptoms, you may need to take additional steps, including consultation with your doctor.

Headaches are categorized according to their underlying causes. Muscle contraction, or **tension,** headaches make up one common group. Vascular (blood-vessel) headaches are a second common category; it includes both **migraine** and **cluster headaches.** A third group consists of headaches caused by **sinus** problems. *(See Sinusitis.)*

Tension headaches, which afflict almost everyone at one time or another, bring on a dull, persistent, non-throbbing pain that can make your head feel as if it's gripped in a tight band. The muscles of your neck may seem knotted, and certain areas on your head and neck may be sensitive to touch. Nerve endings in the head and neck that have been irritated by taut muscles are the chief source of pain. Tension headaches can be short-lived and infrequent, or they can be enduring and chronic.

Migraine is the most debilitating of headaches; it can be completely incapacitating. With some sufferers—a minority—a migraine attack is preceded by a warning sign, called an aura; it may include visual disturbances such as flickering points of light, blind spots, or zigzag lines, or more rarely, numbness in a limb or the smelling of strange odours. Whether a warning occurs or not, a migraine will usually begin with an intense, throbbing pain on one side of the head. This pain may spread and is often accompanied by nausea and vomiting. A migraine can last from a few hours to three days or more and can cause oversensitivity to light, odours, and sound.

All the various symptoms of migraine seem linked to changes in the diameter of blood vessels in the head: the blood vessels constrict during the initial stage and dilate when the headache pain begins. These changes may be due to an imbalance in a brain chemical known as serotonin. Hormones, too, apparently can play a role; there is a strong correlation between changes in oestrogen levels and migraine.

Cluster headaches are so named because they tend to come in bunches. Typically they begin several hours after a person falls asleep and are sometimes preceded by a mild aching sensation on one side of the head. The pain—severe, piercing, and usually located in and around one red, watery eye—is generally accompanied by nasal congestion and a flushed face. It lasts from 30 minutes to two hours, then diminishes or disappears altogether, only to recur perhaps a day later. A barrage of four or more attacks may occur in the course of the day, and cluster headaches can strike every day for weeks or months before going into long periods of remission. The vast majority of sufferers are men.

Sinus headaches are characterized by pain in the forehead, nasal area, eyes, and sometimes the top of the head; in some cases, they also produce a feeling of pressure behind the face. Inflammation or infection of the membranes lining the sinus cavities can give rise to such headaches. Also, the headache pain may stem from suction on the sinus walls, which occurs when nasal congestion creates a partial vacuum in the sinuses.

CAUSES

Headaches strike for many reasons. **Sinus headaches** typically result from hay fever and other seasonal allergies, or from a cold or the flu. With **tension headaches,** stress is the most common trigger; it may stem from anxiety about work or family life, or it may derive from some physical factor such as persistent noise. Eyestrain, poor posture, too much caffeine, or the grinding or clenching of teeth at night can also lead to tension headaches.

Migraine is somewhat more mysterious. Although much evidence indicates that constricting and swelling of blood vessels is involved, some researchers believe that the headaches are primarily neurological in origin. Because migraine often runs in families, it seems likely that genetics can play a role. In any event, a wide range of factors can trigger an attack; among them are excessive caffeine, various foods or scents, naps, dry winds, changes in altitude or seasons,

COMMON SOURCES OF HEADACHE PAIN

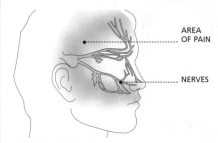

CLUSTER HEADACHE
Although their exact cause is unknown, cluster headaches may arise from pressure on nerves around the eyes. Swollen sinus tissue may press against portions of these nerves, causing these electrical pathways to short-circuit and emit pain signals.

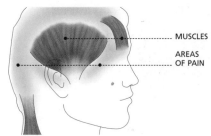

TENSION HEADACHE
Of the various types of tension headaches, one is thought to be linked to disorders in certain muscles in the head and the neck. Pain can be localized around any of these muscles or can spread to affect a broad portion of the scalp.

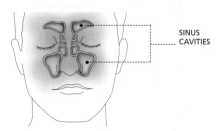

SINUS HEADACHE
With a sinus headache, congestion within the sinus cavities leads to swelling that puts pressure on surrounding tissue and nerves, causing pain to radiate across the face.

ACUPRESSURE

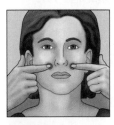

1 Sinus headaches may be relieved by pressing Stomach 3. While looking in a mirror, place the index fingers of both hands at the bottom of your cheekbones, fingertips directly under the pupils of your eyes. Press firmly for one minute. Repeat three times.

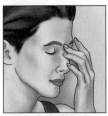

2 Pressure on Governing Vessel 24.5 may help ease headaches. Place the tip of your middle finger at the top of the bridge of your nose, between your eyebrows. Press lightly for two minutes and breathe deeply. Do three to five times, at least twice a day.

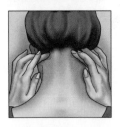

3 To reduce neck muscle stress that may be associated with tension headaches, try pressing Gall Bladder 20. Place the tips of the middle fingers in the hollows at the base of the skull, about two inches apart, on either side of the spine. Press firmly for one minute.

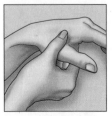

4 Pressing Large Intestine 4 may help relieve sinus headaches. Using the thumb and index finger of your right hand, squeeze the web of your left hand for one minute. Repeat this on the right hand. If pregnant, do not use LI 4.

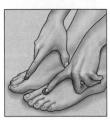

5 Pressure to Liver 3 may provide headache relief. Place the index fingers at the top of each foot, fingertips next to the large knuckle of the big toe, between the big and second toes. Press for one minute, then release. Repeat two or three times, twice daily.

hormonal fluctuations or birth-control pills, missing a meal, or stuffy rooms. Migraine may also occur in the aftermath of intense emotions such as excitement or anger. Exercise, sexual activity, or very cold foods can also jump-start a migraine.

Cluster headaches are the most baffling of all. They are more common in heavy smokers than in non-smokers, and alcohol consumption and certain foods seem to be involved in some cases, but the root cause is unknown.

DIAGNOSTIC AND TEST PROCEDURES

To rule out possible organic causes of headaches— for example, an aneurysm, tumour, or structural abnormality—a physician may employ vision tests, x-rays, a CT scan, a lumbar puncture, or an EEG.

TREATMENT

Both conventional and complementary medicine can be effective in dealing with headaches, and the two approaches may be combined. Almost all practitioners consider **relaxation** beneficial for **tension** and **migraine headaches,** for example.

CONVENTIONAL MEDICINE

Most **tension headaches** can be helped by analgesics such as aspirin, paracetamol, or ibuprofen; antidepressants can help in chronic cases. **Sinus headaches** are relieved by antibiotics and decongestants.

A wide range of medications are prescribed for **migraine.** If you have three or more severe, prolonged migraines per month, your doctor may suggest using prophylactic, or preventive, medications on a continual basis. These include propranolol, a beta-adrenergic blocker that works by reducing constriction in blood vessels; a calcium channel blocker such as verapamil; or antidepressants. If your migraines are milder and occur less often than three times per month, your doctor may suggest drugs such as an isometheptene-containing combination or ergotamine (available as a suppository if the vomiting caused by your migraines prevents you from keeping a pill down). The drug sumatriptan, available in tablet or injectable form, is designed to treat migraine and brings dramatic relief. A therapeutic nasal spray based on the serotonin-inhibiting drug dihydroergotamine acts quickly to constrict blood vessels and reduce inflammation. Even aspirin, if taken in effervescent form at the first sign of an attack, can be effective. Drink it 10 minutes after taking metoclopramide, which reduces nausea and improves absorption, to shorten an attack.

Simple analgesics do little for **cluster headaches,** because they do not act quickly enough. However, doctors have found that inhaling pure oxygen can be highly effective in providing relief. *(See Home Remedies, page 101.)* A short course of corticosteroids, methysergide maleate, and lithium carbonate can alleviate cluster headaches, as can some of the calcium channel blockers and vasoconstrictors that are used for migraines.

COMPLEMENTARY CHOICES

The vast majority of complementary therapies attempt to address the underlying causes of headaches. Because tension and stress so often figure in headaches, relaxation techniques are a staple of therapeutic programmes.

ACUPRESSURE

Follow the illustrations at far left to locate pressure points associated with headache relief. These techniques are often used in combination with one of the aromatherapy oils below.

AROMATHERAPY

The following herbal oils may aid relaxation, easing the pain of **tension** or **migraine** headaches. Moisten your fingertips with one or two drops of lavender *(Lavandula officinalis)* essential oil blended with a so-called carrier oil such as sunflower oil, then gently massage your temples with a circular motion; repeat in the hollows at the sides of your eyes, behind your ears, and over your neck. For a **sinus headache,** try the same techniques using eucalyptus *(Eucalyptus globulus)* or wintergreen *(Gaultheria procumbens).* For any type of headache, inhale a blend of lavender, rosemary *(Rosmarinus officinalis),* and peppermint *(Mentha piperita).* Compresses applied to the affected area or a bath using these oils can relax muscles, easing pain.

CHIROPRACTIC/OSTEOPATHY

Some **tension headaches** are caused by posture that puts unnecessary strain on muscles. A chiropractor may be able to remove the strain through spinal or cervical manipulation and realignment. In some studies, spinal manipulation has been shown to produce fewer side effects and have longer-lasting results than conventional drug use.

HERBAL THERAPIES

Perhaps the most widely recommended herbal remedy for treating and preventing **migraine** is feverfew *(Chrysanthemum parthenium),* which is thought to work by blocking excessive secretion of serotonin, a neurotransmitter. When blood vessels constrict in the initial stage of a migraine, serotonin is released; feverfew may help counteract this by dilating those blood vessels. Chewing a leaf or two daily is one approach to prevention, but this can occasionally cause mouth ulcers; as a substitute for the leaves, you can use 125-mg

C A U T I O N !

Although they can be effective against headaches when used on a temporary basis, painkillers—especially those containing caffeine or codeine—should not be taken over long periods of time. Studies show that the constant use of painkillers may have a rebound effect—actually causing headaches—or can block other medications, such as prophylactic drugs, that you may be taking on a regular basis to prevent migraine headaches. Dependence on painkillers may also hamper the effectiveness of endorphins, the body's natural painkillers. It also seems that dependence on painkillers may permanently alter the pain-control pathways in the brain and spinal cord.

capsules. To offset an acute attack, take 3 or 4 capsules right away, then continue this dosage every four hours; but don't exceed 12 capsules in a day. Migraines brought on by stress may benefit from a combination of equal parts of hawthorn *(Crataegus monogyna)*, linden *(Tilia* spp.), wood betony *(Stachys officinalis)*, skullcap *(Scutellaria lateriflora)*, and cramp bark *(Viburnum opulus)*, taken three times a day as a tea or tincture. For migraines accompanied by nausea and vomiting, try taking 500 mg of dried ginger *(Zingiber officinale)* with water at the onset of the warning stage, if your headache pattern includes an aura; repeat every two hours if needed. Three daily doses of goldenseal *(Hydrastis canadensis)* in tincture, tea, or powdered form may help reduce **sinus headache** pain.

Tension headaches may respond to three daily infusions of valerian *(Valeriana officinalis)* when combined with skullcap and passionflower *(Passiflora incarnata)*. **Cluster headaches** may get quick relief from several daily applications inside the nostrils of an over-the-counter ointment made from cayenne *(Capsicum frutescens)*.

HOMEOPATHY

A range of homeopathic medicines are available to treat specific types of headaches. For a throbbing headache that is worse on the right side when lying down, try Belladonna. For severe, 'splitting' headaches that feel worse with motion, noise, light, or touch, try Bryonia. For **sinus** pain with a thick, green nasal discharge, consider Kali bichromicum. For **migraine** or other chronic headaches, see a homeopathic practitioner.

LIFESTYLE

Regular **exercise** can release endorphins, the body's natural painkilling agents. Exercise may also help to dilate blood vessels, which increases blood flow and may counteract the constricting action that occurs at the onset of most **migraine.**

To nip a **tension headache** in the bud, try the following exercise while breathing deeply and thinking calm thoughts: While seated, inhale and gently tip your head back until you're looking up at the ceiling (be careful not to tip your head back too far, since this can compress the cervical

POURING PAIN AWAY

Your imagination can sometimes be the best medicine for a headache. Try this technique, which relies on your mind's own power to overcome pain. It helps to have a partner talk you through this exercise, but with practice you may be able to do it yourself.

Close your eyes and imagine that your headache is a liquid that fills a certain size of container—the more painful the headache, the bigger the container. Now imagine pouring your headache pain into a slightly smaller container, without letting any of the liquid overflow. Keep pouring the liquid into smaller and smaller containers; bit by bit, you should feel the pain reducing.

spine); exhale and bring your head forward until your chin rests on your chest; repeat twice.

Keeping a headache diary can help you pinpoint the factors causing your specific headache patterns. The diary should provide answers to these 10 questions:

1. When did you first develop headaches?
2. How often do you have them?
3. Do you experience symptoms prior to the headaches?
4. Where is the pain exactly?
5. How long does it last?
6. At what time of day do the headaches occur?
7. Does the eating of certain types of food precede your headaches?
8. If you're female, at what time in your monthly cycle do they occur?
9. Are the headaches triggered by physical or environmental factors, such as odour, noise, or certain kinds of weather?
10. What words most accurately describe the

pain of your headache: throbbing, stabbing, blinding, piercing . . . ?

MASSAGE
Massage therapy can relieve headache-producing tension in the muscles of your head, neck, shoulders, and face. Try giving yourself a 10-minute scalp massage: Place both middle fingers on your forehead at your hairline; using gentle pressure, gradually work them back to the crown of your head; tracing your hairline, repeat this motion in 12mm increments until you reach your temples; rotate your fingers on both sides for a few minutes; then bring both thumbs to the base of your skull along your hairline and massage both sides of your skull up to your crown to release any tightness.

MIND/BODY MEDICINE
Meditation and **progressive relaxation** therapies are effective in reducing stress, which can cause **tension headaches. Biofeedback** training methods can also be helpful in controlling stress. **Migraine headaches,** too, can be treated through a biofeedback method called thermal biofeedback, in which you learn to increase the temperature of your hands and feet. Warming these extremities involves dilating the vessels that carry blood to them—a process that, in turn, may reduce abnormal blood-vessel constriction in the skull and possibly result in diminished migraine frequency, intensity, and duration.

NUTRITION AND DIET
Among the foods associated with **migraine headaches** are chocolate, cheeses, citrus fruits, processed meats containing sodium nitrates or the food additive MSG, and red wine. Keeping a food diary can help identify foods to eliminate.

Magnesium relaxes constricted blood vessels; low levels of magnesium may contribute to **migraine** and **cluster headaches.** Supplemental doses of 200 mg three times a day may be preventive. Taking 50 to 200 mg of niacin (vitamin B$_3$) and niacinamide at the first hint of pain may help keep blood vessels dilated, possibly reducing the initial constriction phase of **migraine** and avoiding an attack.

OSTEOPATHY
Osteopaths believe headache pain stemming from pressure on nerves or blood vessels can be eased by neuromuscular manipulation and soft-tissue massage of your head, neck, and upper back.

HOME REMEDIES
◆ Holding an ice pack or a bag of frozen vegetables against your forehead while soaking your feet in hot water may stop a **migraine** if done right away.
◆ At the first sign of a headache, drink three glasses of very cold water, then retire with a cold compress to a dark, quiet room to sleep (without a pillow).
◆ Inhaling pure oxygen from a tank kept near your bed may offset nighttime attacks of a **cluster headache.** But be sure to consult a doctor on how to use the oxygen. ∎

SYMPTOMS

If your child has measles, he will be very sick. Look for the following symptoms:

- Days 1-3: mild to high fever, harsh cough, runny nose, red eyes, and sneezing; tiny white spots on gums near upper molars or inside cheeks.
- Days 4-8: high fever; characteristic rash, spreading from face to trunk, then to arms and legs. Skin starts to peel in 2 to 3 days. Rash fades from the face by the time it reaches the arms and legs.

Your child may also develop inflammation of the eyes (conjunctivitis), which will make the eyes sensitive to light.

CALL YOUR DOCTOR IF:

- ◆ you think your child has measles; your doctor may have received notice of an epidemic and may be able to confirm your diagnosis over the phone.
- ◆ your child has measles and his cough becomes harsher or more productive, which could indicate viral pneumonia.
- ◆ your child has measles and is having trouble staying fully awake; is extremely lethargic; or is suffering from irritability, disorientation, or convulsions within a week of the onset of the rash. This could indicate encephalitis.
- ◆ your child has measles and develops difficulty hearing or pain in the ears, which may indicate an ear infection.

Measles is one of the most contagious childhood viral infections and one of the most severe, with complications ranging from ear infections to pneumonia and encephalitis (an inflammation of the brain that occurs in 1 out of 1,000 patients). Measles can easily become an epidemic in schools. Preventive immunization is recommended.

Adults can contract measles if they have not been previously exposed or immunized. People who have once had measles develop a natural immunity and cannot contract it again.

CAUSES

Measles is a virus that is transmitted by direct contact or by droplets from a sneeze or cough. The incubation period—when the virus multiplies in the body and the child is not contagious—is 8 to 12 days. Your child is most contagious 2 days before symptoms appear, although he is still contagious for 4 days after the rash begins.

TREATMENT

If you suspect that your child has measles, you should always consult your child's doctor, who will want to notify the schools and will also want to monitor your child's progress so as to be ready to intercede if complications arise. Infected children should not return to school until at least a week after the rash appears.

CAUTION!

Never give your child aspirin—even baby aspirin—or other products containing the salt called salicylate to reduce a fever or to relieve pain. Aspirin has been linked to Reye's syndrome, a rare but very dangerous illness that causes inflammation of the liver and brain.

In the first 24 hours, small, pale red spots appear along the hairline and behind the ears, then spread across the face and down the torso *(right)*; they later spread onto the arms and legs. The spots typically expand into irregular patches.

By the third day, the rash becomes more profuse and pronounced. As it wanes, it may become scaly and take on a brownish tinge. The rash usually disappears within a week.

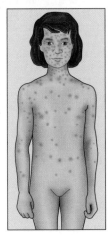

CONVENTIONAL MEDICINE

Your child's doctor will prescribe bed rest, a soft-foods diet, and increased liquid intake. The doctor may also give a gamma globulin injection to family members not previously exposed or immunized. While this won't prevent measles from spreading, it may make the course of the illness less severe for at-risk individuals.

COMPLEMENTARY CHOICES

Do not rely on home treatment alone; consult the child's primary healthcare practitioner.

HERBAL THERAPIES

No herbs treat measles specifically. However, a number of preparations may help alleviate the symptoms. Teas of yarrow *(Achillea millefolium)*, catnip *(Nepeta cataria)*, and linden *(Tilia* spp.) may help reduce fever. An eyebright *(Euphrasia officinalis)* eyewash or a chamomile *(Chamaemelum nobile)* compress may ease sensitive eyes. You can seek help from a medical herbalist.

HOMEOPATHY

Always consult a homeopath for appropriate dosages for children. In homeopathic medicine, Aconite is thought to help a child who suffers a sudden onset of fever; has red eyes; is restless, anxious, or fearful, and sensitive to light. Belladonna is suggested when the child has flushed red hot skin, a hot head and face but cold extremities, and high fever. Pulsatilla may help if your child has a mild fever, is weepy, is not thirsty, and has a creamy yellow discharge from the eyes or nose.

OSTEOPATHY

Gentle, rhythmic pressure applied over the spleen, a procedure known as spleen pumping, may enhance the release of white blood cells into the blood. Seek help from an osteopath.

HOME CARE

◆ Children need to be isolated for most of the time they are contagious. A dimmed room may help if their eyes are sensitive to light; in such a case, limit TV viewing and reading.
◆ Calamine lotion, distilled witch hazel or baking soda baths alleviate itching. Paracetamol may reduce fever.
◆ A humidifier can ease a bad cough. Be sure to use one with a humidistat for the proper amount of mist in the air. Always clean the humidifier thoroughly before and after use.

PREVENTION

Many complementary practitioners feel it is better for an otherwise healthy child to contract measles than to be vaccinated, because fighting the illness strengthens the immune system. However, immunization is recommended, as measles can cause epidemics in schools and the disease can prove fatal. The MMR (measles, mumps, and rubella vaccine) is now given at 18 months, with a booster at the age of 4. The homeopathic version of immunization is not an accepted equivalent and will not provide adequate protection, but some homeopaths will prescribe remedies to ease the potential side effects of the MMR injection. ■

- small, painful, craterlike ulcers that appear singly or in clusters on the inside of the mouth, usually lasting 5 to 10 days. The sores are greyish white or pale yellow with red borders; they may occur on the inside of the cheeks and lips, on the tongue, at the base of the gums, or on the soft palate.
- tingling or burning in the mouth; this sensation often occurs 6 to 24 hours before sores appear.

CALL YOUR DOCTOR IF:

- your mouth ulcers are extremely painful; your doctor can give you medication to alleviate pain.
- the sores last more than 14 days; this may indicate a more serious condition that needs treatment.
- you have persistent multiple mouth ulcers, which may indicate an underlying problem, such as a drug reaction or, in rare cases, oral cancer or leukemia.

Mouth ulcers, also known as aphthous ulcers, are annoying infections of the mouth that may afflict as many as one in two people each year. They appear most commonly in adolescents, whose immune systems are not fully developed, and in women just before the onset of menstrual periods. In fact, women are twice as likely as men to get them. If your parents suffered from mouth ulcers, you have a 90 per cent chance of developing them. Often mouth ulcers occur when you are under stress or run down.

Traumatic ulcers, which are caused by injuries, result in similar sores. These injuries are often caused by rough dentures, a slip of the toothbrush, or hot food.

CAUSES

No one knows what causes most mouth ulcers, or why women are more likely to get them. Their appearance, however, often seems related to stress. Some doctors think that mouth ulcers may result from deficiencies in iron, folic acid, vitamin B_{12}, or a combination. Mouth ulcers may also be caused by an immune system defect, such as a food allergy. Mouth ulcers are not thought to be contagious.

TREATMENT

Mouth ulcers generally go away by themselves, and in most cases, you can safely ignore them. Over-the-counter remedies may help the healing process. Some complementary therapies reduce stress and soothe the inflamed area. If an ulcer is extremely painful or doesn't clear up, see your doctor.

CONVENTIONAL MEDICINE
Many doctors suggest the use of over-the-counter ointments to relieve the discomfort of a mouth ulcer. Look for a medicine that contains glycerin, which protects the sore, and peroxide, which fights bacteria. If your sore does not respond to over-the-counter or home treatment,

your doctor may prescribe a drying medication and a strong painkiller. If you have an infection, your doctor may treat it with an antibiotic such as tetracycline.

If the sore is the result of another medical condition, such as a food sensitivity, the underlying condition should be diagnosed and treated.

COMPLEMENTARY CHOICES

Complementary therapies are aimed both at healing sores and at preventing them from recurring.

ACUPRESSURE

To relieve stress, press Gall Bladder 21, the highest point of the shoulder muscle, midway between the outer tip of the shoulder and the spine. If you do this as soon as you notice a tingling in the mouth, before an ulcer develops, it may help reduce its severity. See pages 138-139 for more information on point location.

AROMATHERAPY

Aromatherapists recommend applying antiseptic oils of myrrh *(Commiphora molmol),* tea tree *(Melaleuca leucadendron)*, and geranium *(Pelargonium odoratissimum).* You may also rinse your mouth four times a day with ½ cup water mixed with 1 drop each of the oils of geranium and lavender *(Lavandula officinalis* or *angustifolia).*

CHINESE HERBS

A practitioner of Chinese medicine may create an herbal formula to strengthen your entire system, heal ulcers, and prevent them from recurring.

HERBAL THERAPIES

To heal ulcers and prevent them from recurring, drink dandelion *(Taraxacum officinale)* tea or take capsules of 500 to 1,000 mg of the powdered root three times a day for six weeks. You may also apply compresses made from teas of calendula *(Calendula officinalis),* goldenseal *(Hydrastis canadensis),* or myrrh *(Commiphora molmol).*

MIND/BODY MEDICINE

Mouth ulcers are often brought about by stress.

Learn to **meditate,** listen to **guided imagery** cassettes, and visualize yourself as a healthy, relaxed person. The most important thing is to find a relaxation technique you enjoy and will keep doing.

NUTRITION AND DIET

If you're prone to develop mouth ulcers, avoid coffee, spices, citrus fruits, and other foods that may irritate your mouth.

If your ulcers are caused by a vitamin or mineral deficiency, supplements of vitamins C and B complex, as well as folic acid, iron, and zinc, may help. If you suffer from recurrent mouth ulcers caused by a food sensitivity, avoid the foods that set off the allergic reactions.

HOME REMEDIES

◆ Rinse your mouth four times a day with a combination of 2 oz hydrogen peroxide, 2 oz water, and 1 tsp each of salt and baking soda. Do not swallow.
◆ Rinse your mouth with milk of magnesia to coat sores.
◆ Try mouthwashes that contain the pain-relieving medication chlorhexidine.
◆ Cover the ulcer with a wet tea bag; the tannin will help dry up the sore.
◆ Use over-the-counter salves containing glycerin and peroxide.
◆ Try stress-relieving acupressure exercises.

PREVENTION

◆ Brush your teeth with disinfecting baking soda.
◆ Eat 4 tbsp live-culture yogurt a day; it contains bacteria that can keep your system healthy.
◆ Avoid foods that are spicy, salty, or acidic.
◆ Take vitamin and mineral supplements C, B complex, folic acid, iron, and zinc. ■

MUMPS

SYMPTOMS

- swollen, inflamed salivary glands located above the angle of the jaw, on one or both sides of the face.
- fever and fatigue.
- in some cases, swelling of the salivary glands under the tongue.
- especially in teens and adults, secondary inflammation of the testes, which is visible, or of the ovaries or pancreas, which is felt as abdominal pain.

CALL YOUR DOCTOR IF:

- you suspect your child has mumps, to confirm your diagnosis.
- your child has mumps and has a severe headache and neck pain; these could be signs of meningitis.
- your child has mumps and has severe abdominal pain and vomiting—symptoms of an inflamed pancreas.
- any teenage or adult male family member with mumps has swollen testes, which in extremely rare cases can lead to sterility.

You will have little trouble recognizing a child with mumps, a mild viral infection that occurs most frequently between the ages of 3 and 10. The telltale sign: swelling on one or both sides of your child's face, above the angle of the jaw. Once your child has had mumps, the child will never get it again, having developed what is known as natural immunity.

Mumps is only mildly contagious; there is little risk that other family members will get sick at the same time. Though mumps is usually a childhood illness, teens and adults can also contract it. The case is likely to be no more severe for an older individual, but swelling of the testes in a teenage or adult male should be checked out by your doctor because of a very slight risk of its causing sterility.

CAUSES

Mumps is a virus and is transmitted through the air in droplets from a sneeze or cough, or by direct contact. The incubation period—when the virus multiplies in the body and the person is not contagious—is 16 to 18 days from exposure. A person is contagious 2 days before symptoms appear and for 9 days while symptoms are present.

TREATMENT

Call your child's doctor to confirm your diagnosis of mumps, as well as to ensure that the physician can intercede if complications arise and to keep your child's medical history current. Children with mumps should stay home from school until all symptoms are gone.

CONVENTIONAL MEDICINE

Your doctor will prescribe rest, a soft-foods diet, increased liquids, and heat or ice on the glands to relieve pain. The doctor may also recommend a paracetamol-based pain reliever.

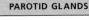
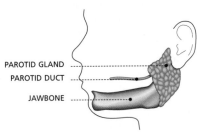

PAROTID GLAND
PAROTID DUCT
JAWBONE

The parotid glands, one of three sets of salivary glands, are located below the ears along the curve of the jaw. They continuously secrete saliva into the mouth through the parotid ducts on the inside of the cheek. When infected with mumps, the parotid glands may swell and become tender to the touch; the openings of the parotid ducts may also contract and prevent the normal flow of saliva.

COMPLEMENTARY CHOICES

ACUPRESSURE
To relieve pain caused by swollen glands, place your middle fingers in the hollows just behind your child's earlobes, and hold lightly for two minutes. Encourage your child to breathe deeply.

HERBAL THERAPIES
No herbs specifically treat mumps, but to reduce swelling, try cleavers/goosegrass (*Galium aparine)* or echinacea (*Echinacea* spp.). Echinacea may help clear the infection. Consult a medical herbalist for dosages.

HOMEOPATHY
Always consult a homeopathic physician for appropriate dosages for children. The homeopath may recommend Belladonna when a child is flushed, red, and has swelling on the right side; Bryonia when a child is irritable, thirsty, and doesn't want to move; or Phytolacca for extremely swollen glands. Stop treatments that don't help within 24 hours; you need to try another remedy.

NUTRITION AND DIET
Offer your child light foods such as soups, veg-

etables, and fruits. Avoid dairy products, which are hard to digest, and citrus fruits or juices, which can aggravate the swollen salivary glands.

OSTEOPATHY
Gentle, rhythmic pressure applied over the spleen, a procedure known as spleen pumping, may enhance the release of white blood cells into the blood. Consult an osteopath.

HOME CARE
◆ Keep your child quiet, especially if he's feverish; confinement to bed is not required.
◆ An ice pack or a heating pad applied to the swelling may relieve pain. A paracetamol-based pain reliever may also help.
◆ A tea made from apple juice and cloves can help relieve painful swallowing. Gently boil eight whole cloves in a good litre of apple juice. Strain and stir, and cool to room temperature.

PREVENTION

Because fighting the illness strengthens the immune system, many practitioners of complementary medicine believe it is better for an otherwise healthy child to contract mumps than to be vaccinated. You should discuss immunization with your child's doctor. The MMR (measles, mumps, and rubella vaccine) is now given at 18 months, with a booster at the age of 4 or between 10 and 12. The homeopathic version of immunization is not an accepted equivalent and will not provide the same protection, but some homeopaths will prescribe remedies to decrease the potential side effects of the MMR injection.

C A U T I O N !
Never give a child aspirin—even baby aspirin—or other products containing the salt called salicylate to reduce a fever or to relieve pain. Aspirin has been linked to Reye's syndrome, a rare but very dangerous illness that causes inflammation of the liver and brain. ■

SYMPTOMS

- redness over the nappy area—around the genitals, buttocks, and thighs, but not on the abdomen.
- tight, papery skin, or skin that is shiny and bright red.
- a strong smell of ammonia.
- in boys, an inflamed penis.

CALL YOUR DOCTOR IF:

- you see no improvement after four days of home treatment, or you also see white patches inside the mouth that appear red after being wiped with a clean cloth; your child may have a yeast infection called candidiasis, or sometimes thrush.
- the rash is scaly and has a yellowish hue and appears not only in the diaper area, but elsewhere on the body, such as behind the ears or under the arms; your child may have seborrhoeic dermatitis.
- the nappy rash does not go away within a few days or worsens; your child may have developed a streptococcal or staphylococcal infection or a local reaction to a particular lotion, soap, or laundry detergent.
- the nappy area is covered with blisters that leave shallow red sores; your child may have impetigo, which requires treatment with antibiotics.
- your son's penis is swollen and red and you can't retract the foreskin, or you notice a greenish discharge from the penis; your child may have a painful condition called balanitis, which requires antibiotics.

Almost all babies develop a nappy rash—an inflammation of the skin on the buttocks, genitals, and thighs—at some time in their young lives. Although a nappy rash may cause a baby discomfort and even some pain, it is rarely serious. Most cases are of short duration, lasting only three or four days. But sometimes a rash will persist, an indication that a secondary skin condition or infection has developed.

Your baby can get nappy rash whether you use disposable or cloth nappy; moisture, not the nappy itself, is the culprit. Keeping your child clean and changing a nappy soon after it is soiled is the key to battling nappy rash.

CAUSES

Nappy rash can be caused by anything that irritates your baby's sensitive skin. The most common source of the problem is urine and stools left in contact with the skin for too long, but a rash can also be caused by inadequate drying of the baby's skin after a bath or by an allergic reaction to lotions or soaps used directly on the baby's skin or to chemicals in the laundry detergent used to clean fabric nappies. Seborrhoea, an inflammatory skin condition that affects the oil glands, can trigger a nappy rash as can thrush, a type of yeast infection. Babies receiving antibiotics for other illnesses are particularly susceptible to thrush-related nappy rash because the drugs allow fungal growth. Eczema, an allergic skin condition, can also occur as a nappy rash in reaction to foods or other allergens.

C A U T I O N !

When baby powder or talc comes in contact with broken skin, it may cause an inflammatory reaction called granulation. If inhaled, the fine powder may cause lung damage. To help keep diapered areas dry, most pediatricians now recommend barrier creams.

TREATMENT

Most nappy rashes respond well to home treatments and require no medical care. If your baby's rash fails to improve after three or four days, see your family doctor, your health visitor or a pediatrician. The rash should be diagnosed to rule out the presence of a more serious infection.

CONVENTIONAL MEDICINE

For an ordinary rash, the doctor may recommend an over-the-counter ointment containing zinc oxide to protect the skin. If your child has developed a bacterial infection, a topical or oral antibiotic may be prescribed. For thrush, the doctor will prescribe an antifungal cream for the rash and possibly an oral antifungal liquid to clear up patches of thrush in your baby's mouth. For nappy rashes involving seborrhoeic dermatitis or eczema, doctors sometimes prescribe hydrocortisone cream. Over-the-counter antifungal and hydrocortisone creams are also available; however, you should check with your child's doctor before using them instead of prescription creams.

COMPLEMENTARY CHOICES

Complementary remedies can be very effective in treating and preventing common nappy rashes. Seek professional medical care, however, if your child's rash does not improve within several days.

AROMATHERAPY

Mix 2 drops each of essential oils of sandalwood, peppermint *(Mentha piperita)*, and lavender *(Lavandula officinalis)* in 4 tbsp of a carrier lotion or oil such as sweet almond oil; gently apply the lotion to the reddened area of skin.

HERBAL THERAPIES

Calendula *(Calendula officinalis)* cream may relieve nappy rash. Herbalists also recommend the following ointment, which you can make at home:

- 1 tbsp each: dried chickweed *(Stellaria media)* leaves, powdered marsh mallow *(Althaea officinalis)* root, and powdered comfrey *(Symphytum officinale)* root.

- ⅛ tsp goldenseal *(Hydrastis canadensis)* root powder.
- 1 cup sweet almond oil.
- ¼ cup beeswax.

In a cast-iron pan, heat the herbs in the oil for 5 to 10 minutes. Don't let them burn. Add beeswax and let it melt. Strain the mixture through cheesecloth into a jar with a tight-fitting lid. Refrigerate until solid. Apply when you put the nappy on your baby. The rash should improve after three or four applications. Discard the cream after two months.

HOME REMEDIES

- At the first sign of redness, wash your baby's bottom with warm water, and dry it thoroughly. Then apply an antiseptic cream and a barrier ointment, such as zinc oxide, to protect the skin.
- Change your baby's nappy as soon as it becomes soiled. Let your baby go without nappies as often as possible.
- Use disposable nappy liners, which allow urine to pass through to the nappy while keeping the baby's skin dry.
- Until the rash clears up, avoid plastic pants or nappy covers, which trap moisture.

PREVENTION

You can't prevent nappy rash, but you can limit its duration or severity by keeping your baby dry and clean and by changing the baby's nappy as soon as it becomes soiled. Wash cloth nappies in hot water (28°C/82°F), use bleach or vinegar in the rinse water, and add extra rinse cycles to help kill bacteria and remove traces of soap. If the entire nappy area is red and irritated, the child may be allergic to your detergent. Try another brand to see if the rash clears. The best preventive measure is to let your baby go without nappies as often as possible. ∎

PREMENSTRUAL SYNDROME

SYMPTOMS

The symptoms of premenstrual syndrome recur during the same phase of the menstrual cycle, usually 7 to 10 days before your period begins. They may include any of the following:

- bloating and fluid retention.
- breast swelling and pain.
- acne, cold sores, or susceptibility to herpes outbreaks.
- weight gain of up to five pounds (from retention of fluids).
- headaches, backaches, and joint or muscle aches.
- moodiness, anxiety, depression, or irritability.
- food cravings, especially for sugary or salty foods or carbohydrates.
- insomnia.
- drowsiness and fatigue, or conversely, extra energy.
- hot flushes or nausea.
- constipation, diarrhoea, or urinary disorders.

A very small number of women with premenstrual syndrome may experience more intense symptoms:

- fits of crying.
- panic attacks.
- suicidal thoughts.
- aggressive or violent behaviour.

CALL YOUR DOCTOR IF:

- your symptoms are severe enough to interfere with your normal functions; your doctor may be able to offer treatments that will alleviate your symptoms.

Premenstrual syndrome—commonly known as PMS—is a physical condition characterized by a variety of symptoms that typically recur during a particular phase of the menstrual cycle, usually a week to 10 days before your period begins. Practically every woman experiences at least one PMS symptom some time in her life, and between 10 and 50 per cent of women suffer from PMS regularly. Specific symptoms vary from woman to woman. Some 5 to 10 per cent of women experience symptoms severe enough for them to seek medical help.

PMS is uncommon in adolescents. Although some adolescents do indeed suffer from the syndrome, for most women the symptoms first develop while they are in their twenties.

Women most often affected by premenstrual syndrome are those who have experienced a major hormonal change, as may happen after childbirth, miscarriage, abortion, or tubal ligation. Women who discontinue birth-control pills may also notice an increase in PMS symptoms until their hormone balance returns.

Although PMS has been reported in the medical literature since the 1930s, its validity as a medical condition is still a hotly debated subject. Some worry that it will be used to prove women too emotionally and physically unpredictable for certain jobs or responsibilities. Experts point out, however, that the syndrome—although sometimes discomforting—is rarely debilitating.

CAUSES

Numerous theories have been proposed to explain some or all of the symptoms of PMS. Many researchers believe that PMS is the result of a hormonal imbalance, although the precise nature of that imbalance is not certain. An overproduction of the hormone oestrogen is sometimes cited; however, most women do not experience PMS at the middle of their menstrual cycle, when oestrogen levels are at their peak.

It has also been suggested that a deficiency in a particular hormone—such as oestrogen, progesterone, testosterone, or prolactin—may be responsible for PMS, but controlled studies have ruled out these single-hormone theories. Recent research has focused on the monthly fluctuations in brain chemicals known as neurotransmitters, including mood-altering endorphins and mono-amines, as a possible cause of the syndrome, but studies have been inconclusive.

Dietary deficiencies, including a lack of vitamin B$_6$ and essential fatty acids, are also considered a possible cause. One type of PMS, characterized by headache, dizziness, heart pounding, increased appetite, and a craving for chocolate, is thought by some researchers to be the result of a magnesium deficiency brought on by stress. According to this theory, the craving for chocolate, a food rich in magnesium, helps balance the deficiency; unfortunately, however, the sugar in chocolate also raises blood insulin levels, which can exacerbate the other symptoms.

The fact that identical twins are more likely to share PMS symptoms than are fraternal twins suggests that premenstrual syndrome may have a genetic component.

DIAGNOSTIC AND TEST PROCEDURES

Before making a diagnosis of PMS, your doctor will want to rule out other possible causes of the symptoms by giving you a general physical and pelvic examination. Some doctors take blood samples to check hormone levels in the body, but many PMS experts consider these tests to be of dubious value. Instead, they suggest that the best way of accurately diagnosing PMS is for you to keep a written daily diary of your symptoms for at least two months. Keep a calendar record of when your menstrual period begins and ends, and each evening write down on the calendar any PMS symptoms you had that day. Your doctor can then use this written record not only to confirm a diagnosis but also to help decide on a possible treatment plan.

TREATMENT

You may decide not to treat your PMS symptoms at all. But if they are severe and you seek help, be aware that some treatment approaches are con-troversial. Remedies for PMS basically fall into two categories: hormonal treatments, prescribed by some conventional doctors, and nutritional and lifestyle changes, prescribed by both conventional and complementary practitioners. Because of the health risks associated with hormonal treatments, many women prefer to try complementary methods first.

CONVENTIONAL MEDICINE

Some doctors prescribe various hormones, most notably oestrogen or progesterone, to relieve symptoms. The hormones are given in a variety of forms, including injection and vaginal or rectal suppositories. But hormonal treatments may produce side effects, some of which can be serious, and no controlled studies have definitively shown that these treatments work.

Some doctors prescribe hormone-containing birth-control pills to women with PMS symptoms. Although some women report that the pills alleviate their symptoms, studies have shown that they are not useful for most women with PMS and may in certain cases even worsen symptoms.

Because of the risks associated with hormonal treatments, many conventional doctors prefer approaches that emphasize good nutrition, regular exercise, and other lifestyle changes such as those described below.

COMPLEMENTARY CHOICES

A wide variety of complementary treatments may help relieve PMS symptoms. Because PMS is different from one woman to the next, you may have to try several treatments, or a combination of them, before you find the right approach for you.

AROMATHERAPY

To relieve anxiety and irritability, try lavender *(Lavandula officinalis)* or chamomile *(Chamaemelum nobile)* oil; parsley *(Petroselinum crispum)* or juniper *(Juniperus communis)* oil may also be helpful. Add several drops to a warm bath.

To relieve breast tenderness, try adding 6 to 8 drops of geranium *(Pelargonium odoratissimum)* oil to a warm bath.

CHINESE HERBS

For relief from PMS symptoms, Chinese herbalists sometimes recommend dong quai *(Angelica sinensis),* which is believed to help balance the body's hormones and have a tonic effect on the uterus and other female organs. Take as a tea or in tincture form (4 to 6 ml) three times a day.

NUTRITION AND DIET

Dietary changes have been shown to effectively reduce PMS symptoms in some women. Try reducing your intake of caffeine, sugar, salt, dairy products, and white flour, which studies have shown can sometimes aggravate PMS symptoms. Many women also find that eating six or more small meals throughout the day rather than three large ones reduces their symptoms, perhaps by keeping insulin levels more constant.

Some PMS symptoms, such as mood swings, fluid retention, bloatedness, breast tenderness, food cravings, and fatigue, have been linked to a deficiency of vitamin B_6 or magnesium. Nutritionists recommend supplements of these nutrients: 50 to 100 mg of vitamin B_6 daily, and 250 mg of magnesium daily, with a gradual increase if necessary. Supplements of calcium, zinc, copper, vitamins A and E, as well as various amino acids and enzymes, are also sometimes prescribed. Consult an experienced nutritionist or naturopath.

Some research has indicated that a dietary deficiency in fatty acids may contribute to PMS. Many women report that taking evening primrose oil *(Oenothera biennis),* a substance that contains essential fatty acids, is effective. Your healthcare practitioner may recommend that you take one capsule (500 mg) daily throughout the month. If this amount does not bring relief, the dosage may be increased to four capsules a day. Other dosage regimens are also recommended. Consult your healthcare practitioner.

HERBAL THERAPIES

Herbalists recommend a wide variety of herbs to help alleviate the many symptoms of PMS. Chaste tree *(Vitex agnus-castus),* for example, is sometimes prescribed because it is believed to help

---

YOGA

A regular programme of yoga throughout the month may help alleviate PMS and cramps.

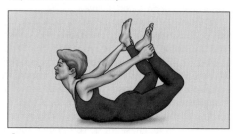

1 To help restore hormonal balance, try the **Bow.** Lie on your stomach, legs bent, and grasp both ankles. While inhaling, squeeze your buttocks and slowly raise your head, chest, and thighs off the floor. Hold for 15 seconds, breathing slowly, and release. Do one time.

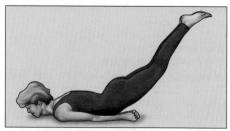

2 The **Locust** tones muscles in the pelvic area. Lie on your stomach, arms at your sides. Squeeze your buttocks as you press down with your arms. Raise your legs, keeping them straight as you press out through the toes and heels. Hold for 15 seconds, then exhale and release. Do once or twice a day.

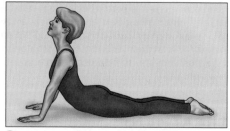

3 You can also try the **Cobra.** Place both forearms on the floor, elbows directly under your shoulders. Inhale and push your chest up while pressing your pelvis and palms against the floor. Hold for 15 seconds, breathing deeply, then slowly relax. Do one or two times.

balance the body's hormones and relieve the anxiety and depression associated with PMS. Dandelion *(Taraxacum officinale),* whose leaves are thought to act as a powerful diuretic, is sometimes used to reduce the bloating and breast swelling caused by premenstrual fluid retention. Skullcap *(Scutellaria lateriflora),* believed to have a calming effect on the nerves, is also sometimes suggested. For an herbal preparation designed to relieve your particular symptoms, see an experienced practitioner.

HOMEOPATHY

For relief from your specific PMS symptoms, consult an experienced homeopath for individualized remedies and dosages.

LIFESTYLE

Studies have shown that regular exercise lessens PMS symptoms, perhaps by stimulating the release of endorphins and other brain chemicals that help relieve stress and lighten mood. Getting enough sleep is also important for the successful treatment of PMS. Lack of sleep can exacerbate fatigue, irritability, and other emotional symptoms. Experts recommend that people who have trouble getting enough rest stick to a regular sleep schedule. By going to bed and awakening at the same time each day, even on weekends, you may find it easier to get the sleep you need.

MIND/BODY MEDICINE

Various relaxation techniques, such as **yoga** and **meditation,** can be helpful in reducing the anxiety, irritability, and other emotional symptoms that sometimes occur premenstrually. The Cobra and Bow yoga positions *(left)* are particularly recommended for PMS.

HOME REMEDIES

◆ Try to eat a low-fat, high-fibre diet. Avoid salt, sugar, caffeine, and dairy products just before your menstrual period.
◆ Exercise regularly.
◆ Try to reduce stress and increase sleep during the week before your period.

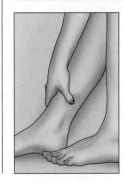

ACUPRESSURE

Symptoms of PMS may be relieved by pressing Spleen 6. Place your thumb four finger widths up from your right inside anklebone, near the edge of the shinbone. Press for one minute, then do the same on the other leg. Do two to three times. Do not use SP 6 if you are pregnant.

◆ Take recommended vitamin supplements.
◆ Try to manage your food cravings—particularly for chocolate; giving in to them may make your symptoms worse. Reach for fruit instead of sugary treats.
◆ As your period approaches, take long, warm baths to ease tension and stress.
◆ Use a hot-water bottle, a heating pad, and electric underblanket, or castor-oil packs to ease backaches and muscle aches associated with PMS.
◆ Abstain from alcohol before your period. It can aggravate PMS depression, headaches, and fatigue, and can trigger food cravings.
◆ Join a PMS support group. Some communities have PMS self-help organizations that meet regularly to provide support and exchange information. Check your phone book or call a local hospital for the name of a group in your area. ■

RASHES

Read down this column to find your symptoms. Then read across.

SYMPTOMS	AILMENT/PROBLEM
◆ scaly, itchy, red rash between the toes; may also cause unusual flaking on the soles of the feet; may affect toenails.	◆ Athlete's foot
◆ rash—either localized or diffuse—in an otherwise healthy person.	◆ Contact dermatitis; allergies; stress; dietary deficiency
◆ rash that progresses rapidly from a simple red flush to small bumps, then a crusted, pimplelike inflammation; extremely itchy.	◆ Chickenpox
◆ red rash in a baby's nappy area.	◆ Nappy rash
◆ tiny pink bumps usually found on the back of the neck and upper back that itch and sting; usually associated with hot, humid weather.	◆ Heat rash
◆ red rash that may resemble a bull's-eye and that fans out several inches from the bite mark; rash is not always obvious; followed by fever, headaches, lethargy, and muscle and joint pain.	◆ Lyme disease
◆ red rash that spreads from face downward and is preceded by fever, cough, and inflamed nasal passages.	◆ Measles
◆ rash that looks similar to the measles rash but is less extensive, lasts for a shorter period of time (usually only three days), and is not accompanied by cough.	◆ Rubella
◆ distinctive red, scaly, round or oval patches with normal skin in the centre; patches gradually get larger.	◆ Ringworm

WHAT TO DO	OTHER INFO
◆ When you bathe, wash and dry your feet thoroughly, and use an antifungal powder. Keep your feet exposed to the air as much as possible. Avoid synthetic socks, tights and footwear.	◆ Tea tree oil (*Melaleuca* spp.) ointment may also be effective.
◆ See your doctor to treat severe cases. Consider mind/body techniques, such as guided imagery, to alleviate stress. Consult a nutritionist; a zinc deficiency may cause a rash.	◆ Stress can play a role as a catalyst for many skin disorders.
◆ Keep a child at home to recuperate and to avoid spreading the disease. Chickenpox is more serious in adults; call your doctor.	◆ The same virus that causes chickenpox can lead to shingles.
◆ For most cases, use an over-the-counter zinc ointment; consult your doctor about more severe or longer-lasting cases.	◆ Nappy rash can be treated with a variety of home remedies and complementary therapies. Changing a nappy as soon as it is soiled will help your baby's skin heal.
◆ Cool your body in a cold bath; wear light, loose clothes in natural fabrics such as cotton or linen; avoid excessive heat; avoid activities that cause you to sweat.	◆ Heat rash is caused by blocked sweat glands. Sometimes it affects babies who are overdressed or who have a fever.
◆ Call your doctor if you think you have been bitten by a tick. Get tested for Lyme disease. Treatment involves antibiotics.	◆ If Lyme disease is not treated in its earliest stages with antibiotics, complications of the heart and nervous system may develop.
◆ Call your child's doctor. Keep your child at home to recuperate and to avoid spreading the disease.	◆ Serious complications of measles include meninigitis, encephalitis and pneumonia.
◆ Keep your child at home to recuperate and to avoid spreading the disease. If you are pregnant and have been exposed to the virus, call your doctor.	◆ The rubella virus can cause birth defects if transmitted by an infected mother to her unborn child.
◆ Try a topical antifungal drug such as miconazole or clotrimazole.	

SYMPTOMS	AILMENT/PROBLEM
◆ light pink, short-lived rash on torso, face, and extremities in children under three years old; occurs three to four days after a fever, lasts less than 48 hours, and does not itch.	◆ Roseola
◆ rash, especially between the fingers and on the wrists, that consists of reddish spots and tiny, grayish lines—the burrows caused by a mother mite digging in with her eggs; extremely itchy.	◆ Scabies
◆ pinpoint lesions on the torso and extremities; raised spots on the tongue; rash peels in five to seven days; sometimes accompanied by fever, headache, vomiting, and chills.	◆ Scarlet fever
◆ painless ulcers on the genitals and sometimes in the mouth, later followed by red, circular, nonitching lesions on the skin, especially on the palms and soles.	◆ Syphilis
◆ bright red rash in a baby's diaper area that does not respond to treatment for standard diaper rash; possibly, white patches in the mouth that leave red sores when wiped away.	◆ Thrush
◆ extremely itchy raised skin lesions with white centers and red rims anywhere on the body; usually part of an allergic reaction to something, such as penicillin or food; extreme heat or cold can also cause an outbreak.	◆ Hives

◆ Allow the rash to run its course without in-nterference from ointments or medication.

◆ Caused by a virus, roseola occurs most of-ten in the spring and fall. The rash usually follows a very high fever (103°F to 105°F). By the time the rash appears, the child is almost fully recovered.

◆ Call your doctor for treatment to kill the mites that cause the disease.

◆ Scabies is highly contagious.

◆ Call your child's pediatrician without delay.

◆ Scarlet fever can cause any of a number of serious complications and can be life-threatening.

◆ Call your doctor. Penicillin in high doses is usually required. Discontinue all sexual re-lations until treatment is completed.

◆ Syphilis is usually transmitted through sexu-al intercourse or oral sex; it can also be transmitted from an infected mother to her unborn baby through the placenta.

◆ See Yeast Infections.

◆ Newborns can contract thrush while pass-ing through the birth canal. It can also be a side effect of long-term diseases, such as diabetes and leukemia, or can appear fol-lowing an aggressive course of antibiotics.

◆ Oral antihistamines may provide relief; avoid applying topical ointments since they may obstruct pores.

SINUSITIS

SYMPTOMS

- feeling of fullness in the face.
- pressure behind the eyes.
- nasal obstruction, difficulty in breathing through the nose.
- nasal discharge.
- foul smell from the nose.
- fever (possibly).
- toothache (possibly).

CALL YOUR DOCTOR IF:

- sinusitis develops into an inflammation around the eye (orbital cellulitis), which could cause damage to the eye and facial nerves.
- the condition does not improve within seven days.
- sinusitis recurs more than three times in a year, and periods between bouts grow shorter; you may have a chronic infection that could become serious.

Sinusitis is an infection or inflammation of the sinuses, the air-filled pockets in the bones of the face. One of the most common healthcare complaints, some researchers estimate that as many as 10 per cent of the country's population suffers chronic (long-term) sinusitis.

Of all the human body's mysterious components, the sinuses are among the most puzzling. Some scientists believe that the sinuses function mainly as mucus factories for the nose and throat. Others say these hollow chambers help warm the air we breathe, still others that they exist merely to lighten the weight of the skull.

All humans have four pairs of sinuses (below, right), which connect to the nasal passages through a series of holes and interconnections. Mucus forms on the surfaces of the sinuses, which are also covered with tiny hairs called cilia. When we breathe, the mucus traps dirt brought in by the air; then the cilia push the mucus out through tiny openings that serve as drains. These openings, known as ostia, are very small, in some cases measuring only a few millimetres across. While the frontal, sphenoidal, and ethmoidal sinuses have ostia at the bottom, the maxillary sinuses have their ostia at the top. Consequently, mucus has to drain upward from these cavities, against the pull of gravity. Given that humans walk erect, it's not surprising that sinus problems are common.

CAUSES

Sinusitis occurs when the mucus-producing linings of the sinuses become inflamed, and by far the most frequent cause of this condition is blockage of the ostia. Once these openings are clogged, foreign material can't get out, oxygen levels drop, and bacteria in the nasal cavity slither into the sinuses, causing the sinus walls to swell and fill with pus. If the infection doesn't go away, the body sends in disease-fighting cells to kill the bacteria. Unfortunately, these well-intentioned bodyguards can themselves do considerable damage to the sinus walls. Defender cells can damage the cilia, the hairlike structures that help expel foreign matter. Furthermore, scarring caused by the cells' battles can result in the formation of sores. Large, mushroom-shaped growths called nasal polyps can also appear inside the nose, interfering with breathing and setting the stage for other problems. Almost invariably, the invading bacteria seek out and colonize adjacent sinuses. More than 40 per cent of all sinusitis patients, in fact, are affected in more than one pair of sinuses.

The most common cause of blockage of the ostia is an upper respiratory tract viral infection, such as a common cold or the flu. These conditions increase secretions in the nasal passageways, provoke swelling of the sinus walls, and cause the cilia to malfunction. Allergic reactions can have the same effect. Hay fever often leads to sinusitis, but allergies to dust, animal dander, foods, smoke, and other pollutants can also trigger reactions that result in blocked sinuses.

In some cases, the ostia are blocked by unusual anatomical features—pre-existing nasal polyps, a deviated septum, foreign bodies, or tumours, for example. Certain diseases, including diabetes and HIV infections, can create a predisposition to sinusitis. And people with poorly working mucus and ciliary functions, such as pa-

tients with cystic fibrosis, have a better than average chance of coming down with the condition. Sinusitis is also common among people with chronic tonsillitis and adenoid problems.

DIAGNOSTIC AND TEST PROCEDURES

In most cases, doctors diagnose sinusitis based on their 'clinical impression', or the sum total of your symptoms, medical history, and the results of a physical examination. Some doctors prefer to verify this impression with a test called transillumination. In this procedure, the doctor shines a special flashlight into your nose and examines the roof of your mouth for signs of sinus congestion. Unfortunately, transillumination might not pick up an infection in a deep, distant sinus. Your doctor may also order an x-ray of your sinuses, but even this technique may not be sensitive enough to detect a deep infection.

Doctors often go ahead and assume you have sinusitis and prescribe medications accordingly. If your body doesn't respond after several attempts, they begin other tests. An ENT surgeon (ear, nose, and throat doctor) may insert a tiny tube into your nose and examine the sinuses directly, a technique known as an endoscopy. A CT scan can show swelling in the deep sinuses and reveal any anatomic abnormalities, but even these scans are not always reliable.

TREATMENT

The goal of most treatments is to open up the sinuses and restore proper drainage. If the sinuses are infected with bacteria, it is important to kill the disease organisms before they cause further damage or spread to other sinuses.

CONVENTIONAL MEDICINE

Before you start treating sinusitis, make sure you actually have it; sinusitis can sometimes be hard to distinguish from an upper respiratory tract infection, dental disorder, asthma, or even a headache.

The bugs that most often invade the sinuses

THE SINUSES

ETHMOIDAL SINUS.......... ....SPHENOIDAL SINUS
FRONTAL SINUS ------ ---- MAXILLARY SINUS

The bones of the face contain air-filled cavities called sinuses. Normally, mucus produced in the sinuses traps debris and drains out through small openings. But if these openings get clogged, foreign material cannot escape. The sinus linings may become inflamed and swollen, causing the pressure, pain, and congestion of sinusitis.

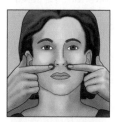

1 Pressing LI 20 may help relieve the pain, congestion, and swelling of sinusitis. Using the index fingers, gently press the points on either side of your nose. Apply pressure upward, underneath your cheekbones. Breathe deeply and hold for one minute.

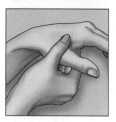

2 To ease headache pain and congestion, try pressing LI 4. With your right thumb, press into the webbing between the thumb and index finger of your left hand. Hold for one minute, then repeat on the other hand. (Do not use if you are pregnant.)

are frequent residents of the nose and throat—*Streptococcus pneumoniae* and *Hemophilus influenzae (H. flu)*. These pathogens usually respond to such tried-and-true antibiotics as ampicillin and amoxicillin. However, because certain strains of *H. flu* have developed resistance to amoxicillin, some doctors prescribe other medications, such as sulfamethoxazole and trimethoprim, cefaclor, and amoxicillin and clavulanate. Other choices are azithromycin and clarithromycin.

Treatment usually lasts 7 to 14 days for acute cases, and from 2 to 3 weeks for chronic or recurrent cases. CAUTION: Stopping the antibiotic treatment prematurely may increase the infection's duration or severity.

Besides antibiotics, many doctors prescribe inhaled steroids such as beclometasone or triamcinolone to reduce inflammation and open the sinuses so they can drain. Decongestants can also reduce swelling and help unclog the sinuses. Most doctors prefer oral decongestants, including pseudoephedrine, over nose sprays like oxymetazoline because sprays can become habit-forming if used for more than three days.

Drugs containing guaifenesin are used to break up hard, encrusted mucus, but they gener-

ally don't work very well. Antihistamines are not usually prescribed for sinusitis because they tend to make mucus thicker and less able to drain from clogged sinuses. Antihistamines may provide some relief, however, if your condition is caused by allergies.

When sinusitis becomes chronic and other remedies fail, your consultant may suggest a sinus washout or surgery. Washout procedures, in which the doctor uses a sterile saline solution to clean out the nasal passages, are rarely performed today. Instead, surgeons prefer surgical techniques such as antrostomy, which involves drilling a hole at the bottom of the frontal sinus to improve drainage. In another procedure, called endoscopic sinus surgery, surgeons insert a tiny scope through the nose. Not only does the scope allow the doctor to see the insides of the nasal cavities, but it also serves to open clogged passageways and remove dead cells from the sinus wall. Between 80 per cent and 90 per cent of patients report moderate to complete relief of symptoms with endoscopic surgery. Extremely rare side effects of this procedure include meningitis, blindness, or double vision.

COMPLEMENTARY CHOICES

Many complementary therapies are attempts to relieve the pain of sinusitis and open the sinuses for drainage. Others aim to fight infection by boosting the immune system.

ACUPRESSURE

Applying gentle pressure to the face and hands can help ease the pain of sinusitis *(see the illustration above, left)*.

ACUPUNCTURE

An acupuncturist will apply medium stimulation to various ear points—adrenal, forehead, internal nose, lung, and near the sinuses—to help drain the sinuses.

AROMATHERAPY

Inhalants of eucalyptus, pine, or thyme may help break up your clogged sinuses. You may also alleviate the symptoms by holding menthol or eucalyptus packs over your sinuses. Other suggestions: Gently swab your nasal passages with oil of bitter orange, or massage your face with essence of lavender mixed into vegetable oil.

CHINESE HERBS

The exact makeup of a prescribed mixture depends on whether the sinusitis is 'hot' (acute or infectious) or 'cold' (chronic or allergic). Either way, the preparation may include the Chinese herb ephedra (Ephedra sinica), a decongestant. (Do not use ephedra if you have hypertension or heart disease.) A number of other Chinese herbs are also helpful in relieving sinusitis symptoms. These include honeysuckle (Lonicera japonica), fritillary bulb (Fritillaria cirrhosa), tangerine peel (Citrus reticulata), xanthium fruit (Xanthium sibiricum), and magnolia flower (Magnolia liliflora).

HERBAL THERAPIES

Bromelain tablets have been shown in controlled studies to reduce inflammation, nasal discharge, headache, and breathing difficulties. You can give your immune system a boost with echinacea (Echinacea spp.), goldenseal (Hydrastis canadensis), or garlic (Allium sativum), preferably raw. Breathing the steam of clove (Syzygium aromaticum) tea or ginger (Zingiber officinale) root tea also provides some relief. To combat excessive mucus production, herbalists suggest elder (Sambucus nigra) flower, eyebright (Euphrasia rostkoviana), marsh mallow (Althaea officinalis), or goldenrod (Solidago virgaurea).

HOMEOPATHY

Homeopaths recommend specific remedies for various types of sinusitis discomfort. For acute sinusitis with thick, stringy mucus and pain in the cheeks or the bridge of the nose, use Kali bichromicum (30c) once or twice a day. For sinusitis with intense facial pain, alternating chills and sweat, and yellow-green discharge from the nose and mouth, use Mercurius vivus (30c) twice a day. For acute sinusitis with a clear, thin discharge, sneezing, headache, and a stopped-up nose at night, use Nux vomica (30c) twice a day. For sinusitis with light yellow or green nasal discharge accompanied by low spirits and lack of

thirst, use Pulsatilla (30c) twice a day. If symptoms linger for more than two days, seek the advice of a professional homeopath.

NUTRITION AND DIET

A good healthy diet including fruits and raw green vegetables can help stimulate secretions and break up sinusitis. Nutritionists and naturopaths also suggest the following supplements to the diet: vitamin C, 100 g per day; bioflavonoids, 1 gram per day; beta carotene (vitamin A), 25,000 IU per day; and zinc lozenges, 23 mg every day for up to one week. Stay away from foods that you suspect may trigger an allergic reaction.

HOME REMEDIES

◆ Inhale steam from a vaporizer, a humidifier, a mixture of hot water and vinegar, or even a cup of tea or coffee. Steam is one of the best and least expensive remedies for unclogging sinuses.
◆ Use warm compresses on your nose to help open your sinuses.
◆ Drink plenty of liquids.

PREVENTION

It's difficult to prevent sinusitis, but you can reduce your chances of having your sinuses become infected. First, avoid allergenic substances. Allergens that people don't often think of include the dust in their beds and certain foods, such as dairy products and wheat. Whenever possible, avoid cigarette smoke. Note: People with diabetes, cystic fibrosis, and certain other diseases may be prone to sinusitis. For help in preventing respiratory infections, see Common Cold and Flu.

■

SORE THROAT

SYMPTOMS

The classic symptoms of a sore throat include a burning sensation or 'scratchiness' in the back of the throat; pain, especially when swallowing; and, perhaps, tenderness along the neck. These symptoms may be accompanied by:

- sneezing and coughing.
- hoarseness.
- runny nose.
- mild fever.
- general fatigue.

CALL YOUR DOCTOR IF:

- ◆ you also have a fever higher than 38°C without other cold symptoms; this may indicate a case of streptococcal throat that needs treatment.
- ◆ you also have flulike symptoms that don't get better after a few days; this may indicate infectious mononucleosis (glandular fever).
- ◆ any hoarseness lasts longer than two weeks; this could be a sign of throat cancer or oral cancer.
- ◆ your sore throat persists for more than a week and is accompanied by nasal discharge; this may be a sign of allergies that require medical attention.
- ◆ your sore throat is accompanied by drooling, or you experience difficulty swallowing or breathing; this may indicate an inflamed epiglottis, the structure that overhangs the opening to the larynx, or an abscess in the back of the throat; these two uncommon conditions require medical attention.

Everyone knows what a sore throat feels like. It is one of the most common health complaints, particularly during the colder months of the year, when respiratory diseases are at their peak. Typically the raw, scratchy, burning feeling at the back of your throat is the first sign you'll have of a cold or the flu on the way. But a sore throat can also presage more serious conditions, so you should watch how it develops, and call your doctor if there are any signs that you have more than the run-of-the-mill type.

CAUSES

At least 90 per cent of sore throats are caused by inflammation of throat tissue, often triggered by viral infections, including the common cold, flu, measles, chickenpox, herpes, and infectious mononucleosis. Bacterial infections, such as pertussis (whooping cough), can also lead to a sore throat. The streptococcus bacterium, which produces the illness known as strep throat, is most commonly at fault, but the bacterium responsible for gonorrhoea can also cause sore throats among people who engage in oral sex.

Living in a dusty or very dry environment can cause a raw and painful throat, as can overuse (or misuse) of the voice, or habitual use of tobacco or alcohol. People who suffer from allergies, persistent coughs, or chronic sinusitis are also prone to sore throats.

In rare cases, a persistent sore throat may be a sign of a potentially cancerous growth in the throat or mouth.

DIAGNOSTIC AND TEST PROCEDURES

If it appears that your sore throat may be the result of a bacterial rather than a viral infection, your doctor may do a throat culture. This painless procedure involves swabbing out a sampling of throat mucus for laboratory analysis. Your doctor's surgery may be equipped to analyse the culture within a few minutes, or you may have to wait a day or two while the sample is sent to an outside laboratory.

For persistent throat pain, or if other symp-

CURING MORNING SORE THROAT

Some people wake up regularly with a sore throat, which then goes away as the day progresses. This 'morning-only' sore throat is often caused by sleeping with your mouth open but can also result from a regurgitation of stomach acids into your throat during the night.

If you think your sore throat may come from sleeping with your mouth open, try a bedroom humidifier or vaporizer (be sure to follow directions for cleaning a humidifier carefully).

If you believe the soreness may be due to a regurgitation of stomach acids, try sleeping on a tilted bed frame. Place bricks or boards under your bed so that the head of the bed is 10 to 15 centimetres higher than the foot. Piling pillows under your head will not help because they will cause your body to bend in a way that will put even more pressure on your esophagus and make the problem worse. Also, avoid eating or drinking anything for an hour or two before going to bed.

toms are present, your doctor may order additional tests to check for other conditions.

TREATMENT

Most sore throats are self-limiting, which means they usually go away on their own without any kind of treatment. In the absence of other symptoms, therefore, you may first want to try alternative treatments for a painful throat. However, if the pain persists or worsens after a few days, you should see your doctor. If left untreated for too long, strep throat may lead to rheumatic fever, which can damage the heart, or to acute nephritis, which can damage the kidneys.

CONVENTIONAL MEDICINE

For a bacterial throat infection, such as strep throat, your doctor will probably prescribe penicillin—or, if you are allergic to penicillin, some other antibiotic such as erythromycin—for 7 to 10 days. To avoid a recurrence, it is very important that you complete the entire course of the antibiotic, even after symptoms have gone away.

Antibiotics are not effective for sore throats caused by viral infections. Your doctor will most likely recommend that you simply rest, drink plenty of liquids, gargle with salt water, and take aspirin or paracetamol if needed for pain relief. Over-the-counter throat lozenges containing a mild anesthetic can also provide relief. CAUTION: Do not give aspirin to a child or young adult with a sore throat, as it may lead to Reye's syndrome, a rare but very serious illness.

COMPLEMENTARY CHOICES

See the illustrations on the following page for **acupressure** techniques that may help relieve the pain of a sore throat. In general, complemetary therapies are geared toward symptom relief, although in some cases they also address the cause of the sore throat.

ACUPUNCTURE

Acupuncture can be very helpful in relieving the pain and reducing the inflammation of a sore throat. A professional acupuncturist will stimulate points along the kidney, large intestine, and stomach meridians. *(See pages 138-139 for information on point locations.)*

AROMATHERAPY

To increase blood circulation and improve fluid drainage in sore areas, massage your throat and chest with a lotion made with 2 drops each of eucalyptus *(Eucalyptus globulus)* and peppermint *(Mentha piperita)* in 2 tsp of a carrier oil such as vegetable or almond oil.

HERBAL THERAPIES

To help fight the infection causing a sore throat, herbalists recommend several herbs with antimicrobial properties. At the first sign of soreness, take three raw cloves of garlic *(Allium sativum)* a day. (Garlic is a natural antibiotic and antiseptic.) If garlic smell becomes a problem, try four garlic oil capsules instead. Teas made from either goldenseal *(Hydrastis canadensis)* or echinacea *(Echinacea spp.)* may also be effective. To make goldenseal tea, pour 1 cup boiling water over 1 tsp powdered herb; let it steep for 10 to 15 minutes, strain, then drink. Repeat three times a day. To make echinacea tea, put 1 to 2 tsp of the root in 1 cup water and bring slowly to a boil; reduce heat and let the tea simmer for 10 to 15 minutes. Cool the tea to a comfortable temperature and drink; repeat three times a day.

Or try a tea made from licorice *(Glycyrrhiza glabra),* which may help enhance the immune system's defenses against bacteria. Put 1 tbsp of the root in 3 cups water; simmer for 10 to 15 minutes. Drink three times a day. CAUTION: Some forms of licorice affect high blood pressure. Use licorice for no longer than one week unless under the care of a health practitioner.

To ease the discomfort of a sore throat, drink teas made from sage *(Salvia officinalis)* or chamomile *(Chamaemelum nobile).* A simple lemon tea can also be very soothing. Squeeze the juice of one lemon into ¼ litre of warm water, add honey to taste, and drink.

Echinacea *(Echinacea spp.)* is one of the best choices for strengthening the body's defences against infection.

HOMEOPATHY

Homeopaths prescribe several remedies for sore throats. Consult a homeopathic practitioner or try those listed here.

◆ If the pain comes on suddenly and is accompanied by great thirst and hoarseness, try Aconite (6c) three times a day.
◆ If the pain comes on suddenly and is accompanied by fever, headache, and restlessness, use Belladonna (6c) three times a day.
◆ If your sore throat has come on gradually and is accompanied by fatigue, try Ferrum

phosphoricum (6c) three times a day.
◆ If the back of your throat is red and swollen and the pain is relieved by cold water or ice, try Apis (6c) three times a day.

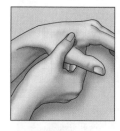

1 For a sore throat from a cold or the flu, try pressing your right thumb into LI 4, between the thumb and index finger of your left hand. Apply firm pressure against the bone above your index finger for one minute, then repeat on the other hand. Do not use during pregnancy.

2 Acupressure may help ease the symptoms of a fever due to a cold. Apply pressure with your thumb to LI 11, located at the outer end of the elbow crease on your left arm. Hold for one minute and repeat on the right arm.

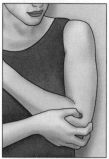

3 To help relieve the discomfort of a sore and swollen throat, try pressure at LU 10. Using your left thumb, apply pressure to the centre of the pad at the base of your right thumb. Hold for one minute and repeat on the other hand.

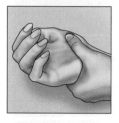

4 To relieve an irritated throat, place your index fingers on SI 17, in the indentations at both corners of your jawbone just below your earlobes. Breathe deeply and press on both sides gently for one minute. These points are very sensitive, so apply pressure slowly and carefully.

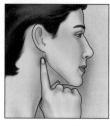

◆ If your sore throat is accompanied by flu-like symptoms, extreme sluggishness, and weakness, use Gelsemium (6c) three times a day.

NUTRITION AND DIET
At the first sign of soreness, take 1 g of vitamin C daily.

Some practitioners of **naturopathic medicine** attribute repeated sore throats to a zinc deficiency. Try a daily supplement of 20 to 40 mg.

If you have frequent sore throats, especially ones associated with ear infections, you may have a food allergy. Consult a healthcare practitioner who specializes in food allergies.

HOME REMEDIES
◆ Get plenty of rest and drink a lot of fluids.
◆ Take aspirin or other over-the-counter medication for pain relief.
◆ Suck on a zinc lozenge—about 23 mg of zinc—every four hours. Zinc can relieve sore throats and other cold symptoms.
◆ To help relieve the pain, apply a warm heating pad or compress to your throat. You can also try a warm chamomile poultice: Mix 1 tbsp dried chamomile flowers into 1 or 2 cups boiling water; steep for five minutes, then strain. Soak a clean cloth or towel in the tea, wring it out, then apply to your throat. Remove the cloth when it becomes cold. Repeat as often as necessary.
◆ A salt plaster may also help provide relief. Mix 2 cups sea salt with 5 to 6 tbsp lukewarm water; the salt should be damp, but not wet. Place the salt in the centre of a dishtowel, then roll the towel along the longer side. Wrap the towel around your neck; cover it with another dry towel. Leave on for as long as you wish.
◆ Try steam inhalations to ease the pain. Run very hot water in a sink. With a towel draped over your head to trap the steam, lean over the sink while the water is running. Breathe deeply through your mouth and nose for 5 to 10 minutes. Repeat several times a day.

HOMEMADE GARGLES
To wash away mucus and irritants and bring relief from the pain of a sore throat, try any of the following gargles:
• **Salt water:** Mix ½ tsp salt with ¼ litre warm water.
• **Sage:** Put 1 to 2 tsp dried leaves in 1 cup boiling water; steep for 10 minutes, then strain and cool until lukewarm.
• **Chamomile:** Steep 1 tsp of the dried herb in 1 cup warm water.
• **Apple cider vinegar:** Mix 2 tsp vinegar in 1 cup warm water.
• **Lemon:** Mix the juice of one lemon in ¼ litre warm water.
• **Horseradish:** Mix 1 tbsp pure horseradish, 1 tsp honey, and 1 tsp ground cloves in ¼ litre warm water.
• **Raspberry:** Put 1 to 2 tsp raspberry leaf in 1 cup boiling water; steep for 10 minutes, then strain and cool until lukewarm.
• **Aspirin:** Dissolve two tablets crushed aspirin in 1 cup warm water.

PREVENTION

If you tend to get recurrent sore throats, replace your toothbrush every month; bacteria can collect on the bristles. Also, be sure to throw away an old toothbrush once you've recovered from a sore throat to avoid reinfecting yourself. Never allow anyone else to use your toothbrush—keep a spare for visitors. ■

TOOTHACHE

- aching or sharp pain in tooth when biting or chewing.
- soreness in teeth, gums, or jaw.

CALL YOUR DENTIST IF:

- your gums are painful, red, and swollen; you may have an impacted tooth or a gum disease.
- you experience continuous bouts of throbbing pain in a tooth, or the tooth is extremely sensitive to heat or cold; you may have tooth decay (a cavity) that requires a new or replacement filling. If the decay is advanced, you may need root canal work. You may also have a tooth abscess, a serious infection requiring emergency treatment.
- you have a sharp pain in your tooth, your tooth feels long or loose, and you have a fever. See your dentist immediately; you may have a tooth abscess.

A toothache can be caused by something as simple as a piece of food wedged between your gum and tooth—in which case relief involves no more than rinsing or flossing away whatever is causing the pain. But if the pain is not so easily eliminated, you probably have a dental disorder that can cause serious problems if you don't visit your dentist without delay.

Tooth decay cannot be cured, but its progress can be halted through conventional dental care. Other causes of dental pain include impacted teeth—teeth that grow at odd angles—and gum disease, which inflames the area around a tooth so much that you cannot tell if the pain is coming from the tooth or from the tissue around the tooth.

Prevention of tooth decay is the best way to avoid toothaches. Complementary remedies may help alleviate the discomfort of symptoms, but conventional treatment is absolutely necessary to stop decay or infection from spreading.

CAUSES

The major cause of **tooth decay** is dental plaque—a substance composed of the bacteria, acids, and sugars in your mouth—which corrodes the protective enamel on your teeth. Initially, you may have no symptoms; but as decay develops, you may feel stabbing pain whenever you eat something hot, cold, sweet, or sour.

If decay goes untreated, bacteria infect the underlying dentine and eventually the pulp, or fleshy core, of the tooth. To fight infection, pus floods the pulp, causing a painful abscess. If left untreated, abscesses can damage the jawbone or sinus and lead to generalized blood poisoning.

Impacted teeth are common in people in their late teens and early twenties, who are getting in their third molars, or wisdom teeth. Wisdom teeth are often too big for the jaw and thus do not fully emerge from the gum or they grow in at odd angles; they press against neighbouring teeth or trap food particles, causing pain and infection.

Toothaches may also be caused by pressure from sinus congestion, by tooth grinding, or by a blow to the face.

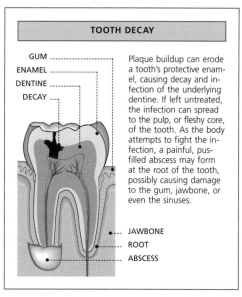

TOOTH DECAY

GUM ....
ENAMEL ....
DENTINE ....
DECAY ....

JAWBONE
ROOT
ABSCESS

Plaque buildup can erode a tooth's protective enamel, causing decay and infection of the underlying dentine. If left untreated, the infection can spread to the pulp, or fleshy core, of the tooth. As the body attempts to fight the infection, a painful, pus-filled abscess may form at the root of the tooth, possibly causing damage to the gum, jawbone, or even the sinuses.

TREATMENT

CONVENTIONAL MEDICINE

For most tooth decay, your dentist will remove the decayed portion and fill the cavity with a durable material. If the decay is serious, you may need a root canal, which involves removing the pulp, sealing the opening, and then capping the tooth with a crown. For abscesses, a dentist will probably first prescribe an antibiotic. If damage is so severe that a root canal treatment is impossible, or if a tooth is impacted, extraction is the usual treatment.

COMPLEMENTARY CHOICES

You must see a dentist for aches that you suspect may be related to tooth decay, but complementary treatments may ease the pain in the meantime.

ACUPRESSURE

Apply deep pressure to the webbing between index finger and thumb (LI 4) to relieve dental pain; massaging this area with an ice cube may also help. Do not press this point if you are pregnant.

HERBAL THERAPY

Rubbing clove oil *(Syzygium aromaticum)* or myrrh *(Commiphora molmol)* on the gum around a painful tooth helps numb it.

HOME REMEDIES

Try the following remedies to relieve your pain.
◆ Rinse with salt water; if rinsing doesn't work, floss gently to pry out any trapped particles.
◆ Numb your gums: Sucking on ice for a minute numbs the gum surrounding a painful tooth.
◆ Keep cool: Though a hot compress may ease pain, if your toothache is caused by an infection, heat will cause the disease to spread.

PREVENTION

◆ Brush and floss after eating; use a non-abrasive, fluoride-based toothpaste. Beware so-called whitening agents; they often contain abrasives that can wear down enamel.
◆ Cut down on sweets and carbohydrates.
◆ Get your teeth cleaned professionally every six months, and make sure a dentist examines your teeth annually.

HYPERSENSITIVE TEETH

If a tooth reacts just to heat or cold, you could have dentinal hypersensitivity. More than 40 million Americans feel pain caused by the wearing away of enamel and exposure of dentine. It's brought on by age, receding gums, dental surgery, or excessive brushing with whitening toothpastes or hard-bristled brushes. You can help relieve hypersensitivity by using a toothpaste made for sensitive teeth and a toothbrush with soft bristles. ■

VOMITING

Read down this column to find your symptoms. Then read across.

SYMPTOMS	AILMENT/PROBLEM
◆ vomiting that appears to be brought on by a specific situation, such as a long car trip or a stressful encounter.	◆ Motion sickness; anxiety
◆ small amounts of vomiting; burning chest pain (heartburn); difficulty swallowing; shortness of breath.	◆ Hiatal hernia
◆ vomiting, headache, nausea; symptoms may be worse with exposure to bright light.	◆ Migraine headache; possibly meningitis
◆ vomiting preceded by intense dizziness, to the extent that everything around you appears to spin; possibly, ringing in your ears.	◆ Inner ear disorder; possibly Ménière's disease
◆ diarrhoea, vomiting, nausea, and fever lasting 48 hours or less, sometimes after you eat rich, spicy, or possibly bad foods, drink an excessive amount of alcohol, or ingest a drug you have never taken before.	◆ Gastroenteritis (also called gastric flu or intestinal flu)
◆ vomiting accompanied by fever, lower abdominal pain, and frequent, malodorous, and/or painful urination.	◆ Kidney infection
◆ recurrent vomiting accompanied by yellowish skin and/or whites of eyes.	◆ Jaundice

WHAT TO DO

OTHER INFO

◆ For motion sickness, ask your doctor about preventive treatment such as antinausea drugs that you can take before you travel. For anxiety, find a relaxation technique— such as yoga—that you're comfortable with and will practise regularly.

◆ Ginger *(Zingiber officinale)* capsules may alleviate motion sickness, as may acupressure.

◆ See your doctor for an accurate diagnosis. Over-the-counter antacids are often the first line of defense against heartburn; avoiding stomach irritants such as alcohol, tobacco, and caffeine can also help.

◆ If you suspect meningitis, **call 999.** Migraine may respond to various analgesics (over-the-counter and prescription varieties).

◆ While meningitis requires emergency medical treatment, symptoms of migraine headache may be relieved by a variety of alternative choices. Herbalists often recommend taking a daily 125-mg capsule of feverfew *(Chrysanthemum parthenium)* to prevent migraine.

◆ See your doctor. You may need antibiotics to clear up an ear infection.

◆ Rest, drink plenty of fluids, and eat bland foods. You may need an antibiotic if your stomach bug is the result of a bacterial infection.

◆ Take care not to let vomiting persist, or your body will lose essential fluids and become dehydrated. To prevent dehydration, drink room-temperature beverages such as water, fruit juice, or soda that has been allowed to go flat.

◆ Call your doctor today. You may need prescription antibiotics to treat the infection.

◆ If you are prone to kidney infections, drinking cranberry juice daily may keep them at bay. Cranberry capsules are also available.

◆ Call your doctor. There are many possible causes of jaundice, and some are serious.

◆ If your skin is yellow but the whites of your eyes are still white, you probably have carotenaemia, not jaundice. Carotenaemia is a harmless effect of high levels of the pigment carotene in the body and can be brought on by a diet rich in leafy green vegetables, carrots, and oranges.

SYMPTOMS	AILMENT/PROBLEM
◆ vomiting accompanied by severe pain in or around one eye.	◆ Glaucoma
◆ vomiting, fever, headache, nausea; unusual sleepiness and/or confusion; possibly, staggering walk.	◆ Meningitis; encephalitis (inflammation of the brain, usually caused by a virus transmitted by mosquitoes); Reye's syndrome (a neurological disorder typically seen in children, which may occur after aspirin has been given for an infection or chickenpox)
◆ nausea and vomiting; whitish bowel movements; dark urine.	◆ Hepatitis
◆ intense, recurrent abdominal pain that is not relieved by vomiting; loss of appetite.	◆ Appendicitis; stomach ulcer; possibly stomach cancer
◆ vomit that smells like faeces, accompanied by constipation.	◆ Intestinal obstruction (the intestines are blocked); possibly, colorectal cancer
◆ headache, vomiting, drowsiness, confusion and/or aberrant behaviour.	◆ Possibly, brain cancer or an aneurysm
◆ severe headache that occurs several hours or days after a head injury; nausea and possibly vomiting; drowsiness, confusion; dilation of one or both pupils.	◆ Concussion (neurological problems caused by head trauma); severe cases may also include bleeding within the skull
◆ vomit containing blood or material that looks like coffee grounds.	◆ Internal bleeding, possibly from a stomach ulcer, stomach cancer, or throat cancer
◆ You are—or may be—in the first three months of pregnancy, and have vomited on several days of the past week or more.	◆ Normal effects (sometimes called morning sickness, though it can occur any time of day) often felt during the first three months of pregnancy

◆ Call your doctor today. Depending on the type of glaucoma, you may need beta-adrenergic blockers to reduce eye pressure or surgery to help the eye drain fluid.

◆ Blindness may occur in as little as three to five days with some types of glaucoma. Early, fast treatment is essential.

◆ **Call 999 now.** Each of these illnesses is serious; Reye's syndrome in particular escalates quickly and can be fatal.

◆ To avoid Reye's syndrome, never give aspirin to a child with fever; use paracetamol instead.

◆ **Call 999 now.** You may need emergency care.

◆ Improved nutrition and a specific diet may help in recovery.

◆ **Call your doctor now.** An accurate diagnosis is essential. Appendicitis requires immediate surgery.

◆ Appendicitis is most common between ages 10 and 30.

◆ **Call 999 now.** Intestinal obstruction can be fatal within hours if left untreated. Successful treatment of colorectal cancer depends on an early and accurate diagnosis.

◆ Scar tissue from a previous surgery is the most frequent cause of intestinal obstruction.

◆ **Call 999 now;** these are serious conditions that may require immediate surgery.

◆ **Call 999 now.** Although a mild concussion may not require medical treatment, there is no way to tell if bleeding is occurring. Bleeding within the skull is a medical emergency.

◆ Prevent head trauma whenever you can by using seat belts in vehicles and wearing helmets for sports such as bicycling, riding, cricket, and ice skating.

◆ **Call 999 now.** Internal bleeding calls for prompt intervention, as well as a follow-up evaluation to determine its cause.

◆ Try not to let your stomach become empty, which seems to make morning sickness worse. Eat soda biscuits or soda bread frequently to prevent nausea or to calm existing nausea.

◆ Vitamin B_6 may help combat morning sickness, but consult with your doctor before trying any supplements, medications, or therapies.

WARTS AND VERRUCAS

SYMPTOMS

- Common warts are small, hard, rough lumps that are round and elevated; they usually appear on hands and fingers and may be flesh-coloured, white, pink, or granulated.
- Digitate warts are horny and finger-like, with pea-shaped bases; they appear on the scalp or near the hairline.
- Filiform warts are thin and thread-like; they commonly appear on the face and neck.
- Flat warts appear in groups of up to several hundred, usually on the face, neck, chest, knees, hands, wrists, or forearms; they are slightly raised and have smooth, flat, or rounded tops.
- Periungual warts are rough, irregular, and elevated; they appear at the edges of fingernails and toenails and may extend under the nails, causing pain.

CALL YOUR DOCTOR IF:

- over-the-counter remedies don't work.
- you are a woman and develop genital warts, which in rare cases may indicate cervical cancer.
- you are older than 45 and discover what looks like a wart; it may instead be a symptom of a more serious skin condition, such as skin cancer.
- warts multiply and spread, causing embarrassment or discomfort.
- you notice a change in a wart's colour or size; this could indicate skin cancer.

After acne, warts are the most common dermatological complaint. Three out of four people will develop a wart (verruca vulgaris) at some time in their lives. Warts are slightly contagious, and you can spread them to other parts of your body by touching them or shaving around infected areas. Children and young adults are more prone to getting warts and verrucas because their defence mechanisms may not be fully developed, but it is possible to get a wart at any age.

CAUSES

Warts are caused by the human papilloma virus (HPV), which enters the skin through a cut or scratch and causes cells to multiply rapidly. Usually, warts spread through direct contact, but it is possible to pick up the virus in moist environments, such as showers and locker rooms.

DIAGNOSTIC AND TEST PROCEDURES

In most cases you don't need to undergo tests for other conditions if you develop a wart. But if you're over 45, your doctor may want to examine the growth, possibly after removing it, to ensure that it is benign.

TREATMENT

Many doctors say that the best treatment for warts is no treatment at all. Most people develop an immune response that causes warts to go away by themselves. One-fifth of all warts disappear within six months, and two-thirds are gone within two years. However, if your wart doesn't disappear, or if it's unsightly or uncomfortable, you can try self-treatment or seek help from your doctor.

CONVENTIONAL MEDICINE

If you decide to treat your own wart, your first-choice remedy should be an over-the-counter medication in liquid, gel, pad, or ointment form.

Most of these contain salicylic acid, the main constituent of aspirin, which softens abnormal skin cells and dissolves them.

First, soak the wart in warm water for five minutes to help the medication penetrate the skin. Then gently rub off dead skin cells with a washcloth or pumice stone. Before applying the medicine, coat the area around the wart with Vaseline petroleum jelly to keep the medicine away from healthy or sensitive skin.

If over-the-counter treatment fails, your doctor can remove a wart by:
◆ freezing it with liquid nitrogen.
◆ burning it off with electricity or a laser.
◆ excising it (a minor surgical procedure).
◆ dissolving it by wrapping it in a plaster patch impregnated with salicylic acid.

Any of these treatments can cause scarring, so instead you may want to ask your doctor about a prescription patch that clears up warts by delivering a continuous dose of medication.

COMPLEMENTARY CHOICES

CHINESE HERBS
A doctor of Chinese medicine may place a slice of ginger (Zingiber officinale) root on top of the wart and cover it with smouldering mugwort (Artemisia vulgaris). The burning herb enables the ginger to release its antiviral constituents. This process is called indirect moxibustion.

HERBAL THERAPIES
Several herbs contain chemicals thought to fight viruses and help treat skin conditions. Herbalists recommend applying the sticky juices of dandelion (Taraxacum officinale), pleurisy root/milkweed (Asclepias syriaca), and greater celandine (Chelidonium majus). An ointment of thuja (Thuja occidentalis) applied four or five times a day may also help.

HOMEOPATHY
Homeopathic medicines for warts include Causticum, Nitric acid, and Antimonium crudum.

NUTRITION AND DIET
To strengthen your immune system, eat dark green and yellow vegetables, which contain vitamin A, as well as onions, garlic, Brussels sprouts, cabbage, and broccoli, which contain sulphur. Supplements to help fight off warts include beta carotene, L-cysteine, zinc, and vitamins B complex, C, and E.

HOME REMEDIES
There are countless folk cures for warts. One that may have some validity is rubbing the wart with a slice of raw potato or the inner side of a banana skin; both contain chemicals that may dissolve the wart. You might also try any of the following applications:
◆ vitamins A and E, which are generally good for skin conditions.
◆ a paste of crushed vitamin C tablets and water.
◆ over-the-counter medicines or a paste of crushed aspirin; both contain wart-dissolving salicylic acid.
◆ aloe (Aloe barbadensis), dandelion, or milkweed juices.
◆ cotton wool soaked in fresh pineapple juice, which contains a dissolving enzyme.

PREVENTION

Practise good hygiene, and eat balanced meals high in vitamins A, C, and E to boost your immune system. Avoid stress, which can compromise your immunity, and learn to relax.

C A U T I O N !

Be sure your growth is a wart. It could be any of several benign skin growths, such as a mole or a corn or callus, but there is also a chance it could be a form of skin cancer. Warts are usually pale, skin-coloured growths with a rough surface. If your growth doesn't look like this, play it safe and see a doctor. Also check with your doctor if a mole or wart's appearance changes. ■

SYMPTOMS

- abdominal bloating and pain.
- belching.
- passing wind.

CALL YOUR DOCTOR IF:

- you have persistent, unexplained bloating for more than three days; you may have a more severe abdominal disorder.
- you have severe abdominal pain; you may have appendicitis.
- you have pain in your upper right abdomen; you might have gallstones or a stomach ulcer.
- you are flatulent and have lower abdominal pain that decreases when you pass wind or have a bowel movement; you may have irritable bowel syndrome.
- you are flatulent, are losing weight, and have pale, foul bowel movements; you might have a malabsorption disorder, in which your intestines are not able to digest fat.

Wind and wind pains are a normal part of your digestive process. People may typically pass wind more than 10 times a day, but you can greatly exceed that average and still be perfectly healthy. You can usually prevent and treat wind and wind pains without professional care, but if you have other symptoms, you should consult with a doctor to find out if you have a more serious health problem.

CAUSES

When air enters your stomach, you may expel it through belching. You can take in air when you eat or drink, especially if you eat quickly. Drinking through a straw, drinking carbonated beverages, chewing gum, wearing false teeth, or swallowing air from nervous habit may also increase the amount of air that gets into your stomach.

If you eat high-fibre foods such as beans, vegetables, fruit, or grains, the partially digested cell walls of these foods will pass into your intestines, where bacteria begin a fermentation process that produces wind. If you have lactose intolerance, you do not produce enough lactase, a digestive enzyme that breaks down milk sugars, and you are more likely to produce gas after eating dairy foods. A gastrointestinal infection may also produce intestinal wind.

TREATMENT

You can usually treat wind and wind pains without the active involvement of a healthcare professional. Conventional medicine suggests decreasing excessive wind through changes in diet and use of over-the-counter preparations. Complementary medicines offer a wide variety of treatments.

CONVENTIONAL MEDICINE

A doctor will probably suggest you treat wind problems by changing what you eat. Avoid high-fibre foods like beans, milk products, alcohol, and carbonated beverages. Moderate exercise after meals can help move wind through your system more quickly. You may also decide to try over-the-counter preparations for wind pains. Simethicone, the active ingredient in most of these over-the-counter preparations, appears to help break up wind bubbles in the large intestine. Activated charcoal tablets absorb intestinal gas, but check with your doctor before using them, because they also absorb medications. If you are lactose intolerant, lactase supplements can help you to digest milk products more effectively. An over-the-counter product containing alpha-galactosidase may reduce the wind that is produced in digesting beans.

COMPLEMENTARY CHOICES

There are many complementary therapies for gas problems. Most of them can be practised at home, but you should check with a practitioner to make sure a particular therapy is suitable for your needs.

ACUPRESSURE

Pressing the following points may help to alleviate gas pains: Conception Vessel 6, Large Intestine 4, Spleen 6, and Stomach 36. *(See pages 8-9 for information on point locations.)*

ACUPUNCTURE

A practitioner can provide treatment for wind using the same points used in acupressure except for Conception Vessel 8, where heat might be applied instead.

HERBAL THERAPIES

Anise water, made by steeping 1 tsp of aniseeds in 1 cup of water for 10 minutes, may be helpful. Teas made with peppermint *(Mentha piperita)*, chamomile *(Chamaemelum nobile)*, or fennel *(Foeniculum vulgare)* may also relieve wind pains.

HOMEOPATHY

Carbo vegetabilis is the most commonly used homeopathic remedy, but Lycopodium is used as well. Nux vomica is used for wind associated with constipation, and Chamomilla is preferred for wind in infants. Talk to a homeopath about which is most suitable for you.

LIFESTYLE

Regular exercise stimulates digestion and promotes the reabsorption and expulsion of wind.

MIND/BODY MEDICINE

Biofeedback and **chi kung** can relieve stress and reduce gas production.

NUTRITION AND DIET

Increase your fibre intake slowly and try avoiding beans, peas, and fermented foods such as cheese, soy sauce, and alcohol. Asafetida powder dispels intestinal wind and may be used as a spice with beans. Drink fewer carbonated drinks. Avoid mixing proteins and carbohydrates at the same meal. Do not overeat, and eat fewer different food items at one sitting. For people who are lactose intolerant, replacing cow's milk with soy milk may help.

REFLEXOLOGY

Stimulate stomach areas to encourage stomach digestion, liver area to trigger bile secretion, gallbladder area to trigger release of stored bile, intestine areas to stimulate regular contractions in both intestines, and pancreas area to encourage secretion of digestive enzymes.

HOME REMEDIES

◆ Drink at at least 10 glasses of water every day.
◆ Walk each day for 15 to 20 minutes.

PREVENTION

One of the main methods of preventing gas and gas pains is also the primary treatment: Avoid foods that generate gas in your system. Try to become more aware of the air that you swallow; you can avoid some gas, for instance, by not gulping your food. Take more exercise. ∎

SYMPTOMS

- painless white patches in your mouth or throat that may come off when you eat or brush your teeth; this indicates **oral thrush,** most common in infants, the elderly, and AIDS patients.
- white patches in the mouth and throat, sometimes associated with painful swallowing; these are symptomatic of **oesophageal thrush,** a potential complication of AIDS.
- peeling skin on the hands, especially between the fingers, and swollen nail folds above the cuticle; possibly painful, red, and containing pus.
- itchy or burning shiny, pink rash with a scaly or blistered edge in the folds of the skin. This indicates **intertrigo.**
- in women, vaginal itching and irritation; redness and swelling of the vulva; unusually thick, white discharge; and pain during intercourse. These are signs of a **vaginal yeast infection,** also known as **candida albicans** or thrush.
- in men, red patches and blisters at the end of the penis and around the foreskin, possibly accompanied by severe itching and pain. These are symptoms of **balanitis.**

CALL YOUR DOCTOR IF:

- you have any of the symptoms for the first time; you need a professional evaluation before beginning treatment.
- the infection does not respond to treatment or recurs; you may have a more serious disorder such as diabetes or an HIV infection.

Yeast, or fungal, infection—sometimes called **candidiasis**—takes many forms. Yeast infections often develop where a moist environment encourages fungal growth, especially on the webs of fingers and toes, nails, genitals, and folds of skin. **Oral thrush** is a painless, often recurrent infection of the mouth and throat; it is common in babies, young children, and the elderly, but can affect all ages. **Candida albicans** or vaginal thrush is a painful vaginal yeast infection experienced by many women, most commonly during pregnancy or treatment with antibiotics. **Balanitis** is a less common but equally irritating infection of the penis. **Systemic yeast infections** can occur in cases of diabetes, AIDS, and other ailments or drug treatments that suppress the immune system.

CAUSES

Candida albicans is a fungal organism, or yeast, that thrives in your mouth, gastrointestinal tract, and skin; your body produces bacterial flora that keeps it in check. When fungal growth exceeds the body's ability to control it, yeast infection develops. This can happen when you are weakened by illness or upset by stress. Modern antibiotics that treat many ailments can kill the bacteria that otherwise control fungal outbreaks.

Yeast infections are common among people whose hands are often in water, in children who suck their thumbs or fingers, and in people whose clothing (synthetics) retains body moisture. The nappy rash called **candidal dermatitis** is caused by yeast growth in the folds of a baby's skin. Diabetics are especially prone to yeast infections because they have high levels of sugar in their blood and urine and a low resistance to infection—conditions that encourage yeast growth. In rare cases the candida fungus may invade the bloodstream through an intravenous (IV) tube or urinary catheter. If the infection travels to the kidneys, lungs, brain, or other organs, it can cause serious systemic complications, but these develop only in people who are seriously ill or who have other health problems that weaken the immune system, such as drug addiction or diabetes.

DIAGNOSTIC AND TEST PROCEDURES

To diagnose **oral thrush,** a doctor will examine the white patches and may take a sample for testing. To check for **vaginal yeast infection,** a doctor may take a vaginal wet smear or swab. If your doctor thinks you have a **systemic yeast infection,** a blood, stool, or tissue sample will be tested for the fungus.

TREATMENT

Treatment will depend on your specific condition but will focus on counteracting the growth of the yeast organism that causes the infection.

CONVENTIONAL MEDICINE

Your doctor will probably treat **oral thrush** with an antifungal medication such as clotrimazole or ketoconazole. Babies with oral thrush are typically given nystatin with a dropper. Infections of the skin or nails can be treated with topical applications of clotrimazole. For **vaginal yeast infection,** an over-the-counter intravaginal cream containing miconazole or clotrimazole is typically suggested. If over-the-counter medications are not effective, your doctor may prescribe a cream with terconazole or an oral antifungal drug such as Diflucan containing fluconazole. If your doctor determines that you have a **systemic yeast infection,** you may get intravenous doses of amphotericin or flucytosine.

COMPLEMENTARY CHOICES

Complementary remedies can strengthen the immune system to resist yeast infections, and can treat specific yeast infections and prevent recurrence.

HERBAL THERAPIES

For healing yeast infections on your skin, apply full-strength tea tree oil (*Melaleuca* spp.) two to three times daily; a slight burning sensation is normal, but discontinue if the treatment is painful. An over-the-counter salve containing

---

CHRONIC YEAST INFECTION

Although the diagnosis is not universally accepted, some doctors recognize a condition called chronic candidiasis, or chronic yeast infection, that may affect the gastrointestinal, nervous, endocrine, and immune systems. Treatment focuses on eliminating predisposing factors, such as prescription or over-the-counter drugs, foods with high refined-sugar or yeast content, high-carbohydrate vegetables, and milk products. Your doctor may also test you for underlying conditions, such as diabetes or thyroid problems.

An herbal remedy for chronic yeast infection is tea brewed from 1 to 2 grams of dried root of barberry (Berberis vulgaris) or goldenseal (Hydrastis canadensis) in a cup of boiling water, taken three times a day. With your doctor's approval, you may want to try taking daily supplements of 45 mg iron, 45 mg zinc, and 200 mcg selenium (avoid higher doses of selenium).

---

marigold/calendula *(Calendula officinalis)* is good for rashes in children over two years of age.

HOMEOPATHY

Numerous homeopathic remedies are used to treat yeast infections; ask a licensed homeopath about which one best suits your symptoms.

PREVENTION

- ◆ If work keeps your hands in water for long periods, wear rubber gloves. When you've finished, wash your hands and apply a mild prescription or over-the-counter antifungal cream.
- ◆ Wear cotton or silk underpants which, unlike nylon and other synthetics, allow excess moisture to evaporate. Wash and dry your underpants thoroughly; change them at least daily. ■

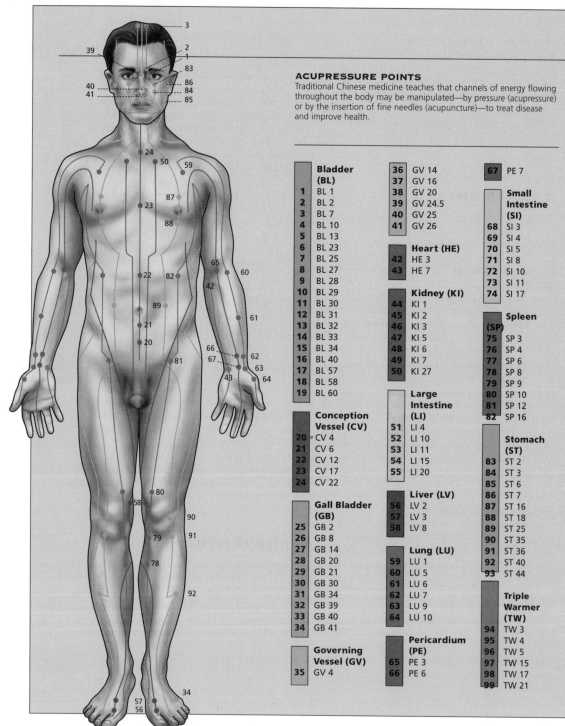

ACUPRESSURE POINTS

Traditional Chinese medicine teaches that channels of energy flowing throughout the body may be manipulated—by pressure (acupressure) or by the insertion of fine needles (acupuncture)—to treat disease and improve health.

Bladder (BL)
1 BL 1
2 BL 2
3 BL 7
4 BL 10
5 BL 13
6 BL 23
7 BL 25
8 BL 27
9 BL 28
10 BL 29
11 BL 30
12 BL 31
13 BL 32
14 BL 33
15 BL 34
16 BL 40
17 BL 57
18 BL 58
19 BL 60

Conception Vessel (CV)
20 CV 4
21 CV 6
22 CV 12
23 CV 17
24 CV 22

Gall Bladder (GB)
25 GB 2
26 GB 8
27 GB 14
28 GB 20
29 GB 21
30 GB 30
31 GB 34
32 GB 39
33 GB 40
34 GB 41

Governing Vessel (GV)
35 GV 4

36 GV 14
37 GV 16
38 GV 20
39 GV 24.5
40 GV 25
41 GV 26

Heart (HE)
42 HE 3
43 HE 7

Kidney (KI)
44 KI 1
45 KI 2
46 KI 3
47 KI 5
48 KI 6
49 KI 7
50 KI 27

Large Intestine (LI)
51 LI 4
52 LI 10
53 LI 11
54 LI 15
55 LI 20

Liver (LV)
56 LV 2
57 LV 3
58 LV 8

Lung (LU)
59 LU 1
60 LU 5
61 LU 6
62 LU 7
63 LU 9
64 LU 10

Pericardium (PE)
65 PE 3
66 PE 6

67 PE 7

Small Intestine (SI)
68 SI 3
69 SI 4
70 SI 5
71 SI 8
72 SI 10
73 SI 11
74 SI 17

Spleen (SP)
75 SP 3
76 SP 4
77 SP 6
78 SP 8
79 SP 9
80 SP 10
81 SP 12
82 SP 16

Stomach (ST)
83 ST 2
84 ST 3
85 ST 6
86 ST 7
87 ST 16
88 ST 18
89 ST 25
90 ST 35
91 ST 36
92 ST 40
93 ST 44

Triple Warmer (TW)
94 TW 3
95 TW 4
96 TW 5
97 TW 15
98 TW 17
99 TW 21

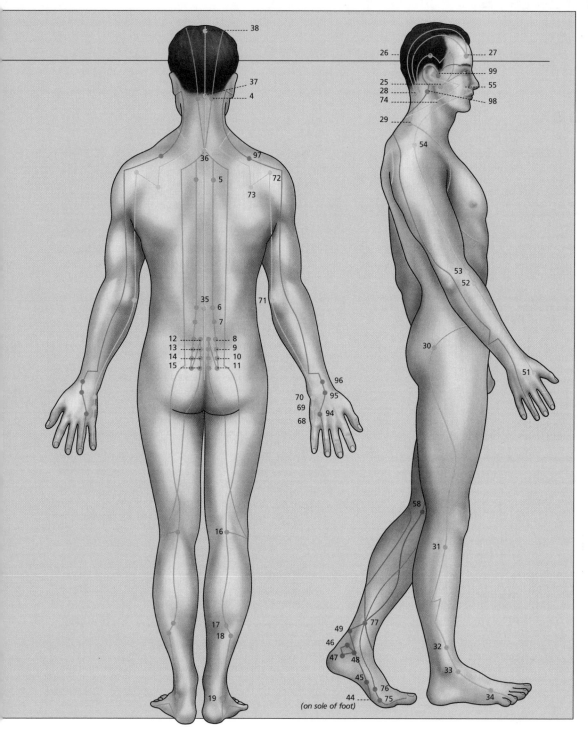

(on sole of foot)

STOCKISTS

East West Herbs 01608 658862
Neal's Yard 020 7498 1686
The Society of Homeopaths 01604 621400
The National Institute of Medical Herbalists 01392 426022

INDEX